Curly Kids

The Handbook

How to Care for Your Child's Glorious Hair

LORRAINE MASSEY

with Michele Bender

WORKMAN PUBLISHING

NAPA COUNTY LIBRARY
580 COOMBS STREET
NAPA, CA 94559

In memory of my dad, Donald Massey,
my brother John Massey,
Elizabeth Cantor, and Francis Delahoz.
And to my forever loves Kaih, Shey,
Dylan, Veronica, Venaih, and Silas

ॐ

Copyright © 2020 by Lorraine Massey and Michele Bender
CG Method and Curl By Curl are trademarked by Lorraine Massey

All rights reserved. No portion of this book may be reproduced—mechanically, electronically,
or by any other means, including photocopying—without written permission of the publisher.
Published simultaneously in Canada by Thomas Allen & Son Limited.

Library of Congress Cataloging-in-Publication Data is available.
ISBN 978-1-5235-0740-5

Design by Becky Terhune
Original photography by Lucy Schaeffer
Author photos: Jeremy Salgada (Lorraine Massey); Adriana Lepetrone (Michelle Bender)
Additional photo credits: Getty Images: Gary Gershoff/Getty Images Entertainment, p. 114.
Shutterstock.com: Makovsky Art, p. 34; Vitawin, p. 40; Tatyana Vyc, p. 165; Miss Treechada Yoksan, p. 66.

Workman books are available at special discounts when purchased in bulk
for premiums and sales promotions as well as for fund-raising or educational use.
Special editions or book excerpts can also be created to specification.
For details, contact the Special Sales Director at the address below or
send an email to specialmarkets@workman.com.

Workman Publishing Co., Inc.
225 Varick Street
New York, NY 10014-4381
workman.com

WORKMAN is a registered trademark of Workman Publishing Co., Inc.

Printed in China
First printing July 2020

10 9 8 7 6 5 4 3 2 1

OCT 1 3 2020

Curly Kids

The Handbook

NAPA COUNTY LIBRARY
580 COOMBS STREET
NAPA, CA 94559

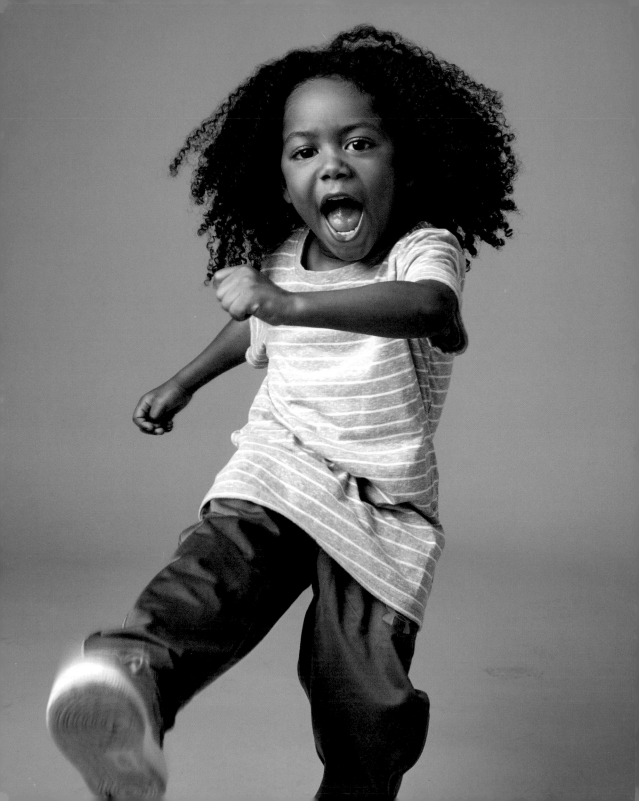

Contents

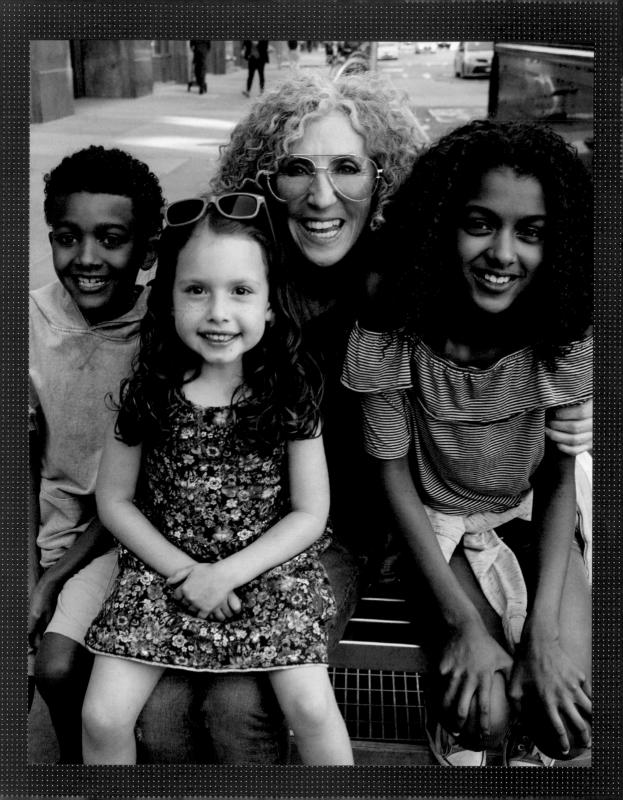

Introduction

Born Free

Curls are like a box of chocolates. You never know what you're gonna get.

~~~~~~~~~~~~~~~~~~~~~~~~~~~~~~~~~~~~~

The goal of *Curly Kids* is to instill an awareness of and healthy connection to the hair we were born with, from infancy through the teen years. Why? Because if we do that, then embracing our natural texture will become a habit and part of our lifestyle. Many curlies can attest that in time, this acceptance of their hair trickles down to other areas of their lives, such as their confidence and self-esteem. Imagine loving your curls from day one! Yes, *loving* them! How is that possible? If you care for curly hair properly from a young age, you won't want to subject it to heat tools, chemical treatments, brushes, and sulfate- and silicone-filled products, among other things, so it will be healthier. In turn, healthier curls are more beautiful curls, making this hair type even *more* accepted and coveted the world over. As a result, this will help even *more* curlies embrace the hair they were born with, no matter their age. As I tell parents: Teach curly kids how to blow-dry or flat-iron their hair and they may be happy for a day (unless it rains). Teach them to love their curls and they will be happy for life!

We know that accepting ourselves without prejudice—honestly and authentically, and sooner rather than later—can be life changing. And who doesn't want self-acceptance for themselves and the people they love, starting now? When we accept

On the surface, *Curly Kids* is a book about hair. But it's also a book about empowering your child, because how you feel about your hair, like most things, is more than skin deep.

ourselves, the positive repercussions for the world are endless. Plus, if our children don't have to put energy into hiding, straightening, lamenting, and worrying about their hair, they can spend their time doing meaningful things, finding true happiness and passion, and changing our world. That freedom is priceless.

When the children in your life are young, you are their curly guardian, so I appreciate you taking the time to better understand their hair—and perhaps your own. Honoring and caring for your child's curls will teach him or her to do the same. Loving the hair you have and knowing how to care for it are not always obvious or encouraged by our society, but it's not hard to learn how to give it the TLC it needs. In fact, nurturing your child's curls is quite simple, and *Curly Kids* will show you the way— from cleansing to cutting and more.

Many curly adults I know grew up with the message that their hair was not acceptable. Often this was because their parents didn't know how to manage it. I'm not placing blame. If they had known better, they would have done better. After all, when we don't understand something, we often ignore it or hide it in hopes of controlling it. Loving and cherishing your curls is a relatively new idea.

Many curly adults have unpleasant childhood memories. They talk about straight-haired moms who didn't know any better and painfully brushed their "knotty" strands—or cut them off completely. Others were teased for having a halo of frizz or endlessly longed for a friend's silky, straight strands and smooth, swinging ponytail. Perhaps, as a rite of passage (often as early as four years old), he or she was taken to a salon (or an aunt's or grandma's kitchen) to have their coils chemically relaxed or altered by a hot comb. These hair stories are endless in number, varied in detail, and come from all cultures and nationalities, but one thing is the same: Many adult curlies say they've tried everything and anything to get smoother hair, including carcinogenic chemicals, blow-frying (my term for blow-drying), flat irons, and spiky bristle rollers. Some curlies growing up in the 1960s wrapped their wet hair around frozen orange juice cans at night and attempted to sleep sitting upright to keep these makeshift curlers in place. Some say they even used a clothing iron on their hair. Besides damaged hair and burns from hot combs or flat irons, they endured damage to their self-esteem. Others have receding hairlines and bald spots and suffered sore, tender scalps and terrible headaches from too much tugging while heat-styling or wearing tightly pulled braids and ponytails.

The good news is that today natural textures are far more accepted than they used to be and not seen as something to be fixed, tamed, or hidden. That was the goal of our first book, *Curly Girl: The Handbook*, which provides advice and techniques on loving and caring for curly hair. In that book, we introduced the Curly Girl/Guy Method (otherwise known as the CG Method™). We've also watched a grassroots movement with one curly girl or guy providing inspiration to another, passing along tips and insights. Still, despite all the curl information that has been disseminated over the last twenty years, plenty of frustration and confusion remain, and learning to love your curly hair can still be a struggle.

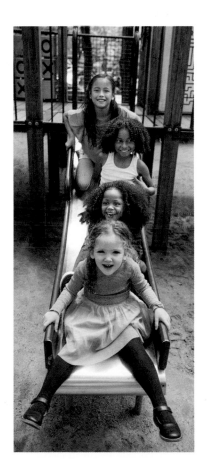

Today, hair-straightening and curl extermination is a billion-dollar industry that capitalizes on the vulnerability of curlies by promising to eradicate, combat, control, smooth, tame, and fight your natural hair texture. The

A STRAIGHT LYE

Hair straightening can be traced way back to the early 1900s. In 1909, Garrett Augustus Morgan, a tailor and inventor, accidentally created straightening cream when he was trying to find a solution to ease friction created by sewing machine needles. While experimenting with this chemical solution, Morgan noticed that the hairs on the wool fabric he was sewing became straighter. (I've always said that hair is like a fine fiber!) After testing the solution on a neighbor's dog's fur and then on himself, he created a company and began selling this straightening cream to African American women. This made Morgan a financial success. After experiencing hair loss and a scalp condition from the lye, one of his customers, Annie Malone, developed her own product, influenced by her aunt, who was an herbalist. But the damage didn't stop there. Madam C. J. Walker used Malone's products and techniques before inventing her own line that made her one of the first female, African American self-made millionaires. Walker went door-to-door telling women of color that her products would help their hair have that "European texture."

manufacturers of these products perpetuate the notion that you can't possibly love the hair you have. In the past, ads have even suggested that hair can be "grown straight"! But that's not possible. Instead, the chemicals in those products leave hair dull, lethargic, and damaged. Years ago, *Allure* magazine published an article called "Scared Straight" about the dangers of the popular Brazilian straightening treatment and detailed the frightening things women will attempt in their quest to have straight hair. The whole piece gave me chills! In it, two women and their hairstylist wear $700 military-grade rubber gas masks to keep from inhaling the chemicals' potent and unhealthy fumes. Plus, one of the treatment's ingredients, formaldehyde, is classified as a human carcinogen by the International Agency for Research on Cancer, part of the World Health Organization. After the article ran, the sales of these treatments went *up*, because many curlies are so desperate to control their coils that this serious health caution didn't matter. Within weeks of applying these caustic solutions, the natural curly roots appear, and the only way to erase them is to repeat the chemical treatment. To me, this is similar to gardeners using a toxic weed killer on a blooming rose garden. Then you are caught in an unhealthy, vicious cycle that is highly addictive, time-consuming, and expensive, which is why Chris Rock called hair-relaxing products "creamy crack" in his movie *Good Hair*.

> A new client told me that her hair was falling out after her last Brazilian straightening treatment. I replied, "I would leave you, too, if I was treated that way!"

Self-acceptance is very important to me, not just because of the painful childhood memories so many curlies have shared with me, but because I have my own curly hair history. Before I knew better, I saw my curls like an arranged marriage—something I wouldn't have chosen, but here we were, till death do us part. And like so many forced relationships, we were destined to experience turbulence, with many storms and crashing waves. I hated my curls from the moment I was able to look in the mirror. And I wasn't the only one who felt this way. In the poor factory town of Leicester, England, where I grew up, curly hair was abhorred much more than it was accepted—especially in my own home. My six brothers and sisters had smooth, straight hair. I, on the other hand, had wild, knotty, corkscrew curls that stuck out all over my head. Think Little Orphan Annie after going through a wind tunnel. For years, I was sure that there'd been some mix-up at the hospital and I'd been sent home with the wrong set of parents. *How could I be curly when they're all straight?* I wondered. I tried to forget how different I was from my siblings, but they reminded me with their relentless teasing.

I remember being as wild as my hair, playing outside and hearing one of my siblings yell, "Get her inside." They didn't want anyone to see me and my untamed tresses, runny nose, mismatched shoes, and

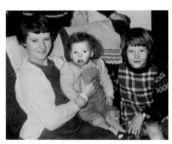

I was a curly toddler.

scruffy clothes. Perhaps my mother felt like it reflected badly on her and gave people the impression she was not taking care of me. My mum tried her best to "tame the wild" by harshly brushing my curls, but this only emphasized the very thing she was trying to control. Her frustration with me was obvious. In my mind, the equation was simple: Straight hair was beautiful; curly was ugly. (However, it wasn't lost on me that fairy tales raved about curls if they were golden and belonged to very young children, although they'd better straighten themselves by the time the children grew up!)

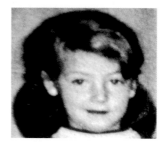

Bright-eyed and brushed-out, 7 years old

Even when I was very young, I was aware of how much I hated my hair. I would often slip a shirt halfway over my head so that it hung down across my back, mimicking what I thought was the feeling of smooth strands. Then I'd stand in front of the mirror with a brush as a microphone, imitating rock stars I'd seen on TV swinging their shiny, stick-straight hair back and forth. I longed to run my fingers effortlessly through my phantom straight strands and feel them move *with* me, not against me. Perhaps that is why, for my fourth birthday, I begged my mother for a straight-haired wig and a grass skirt so I could pretend I was a Polynesian hula dancer. Although we were poor, my mom found a way to get them for me. We had

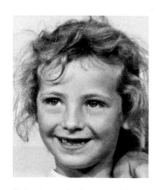

Puberty curls, 9 years old

no electricity that night, just the light of the fireplace, but I have a vivid memory of dancing and pretending to be someone else, with the most joy I had known to that point. That wig, which I wore all day, every day, and the feeling of "hair" swaying down my back, was what sparked the chase for straight hair that lasted for years. I imagine this is today's version of what happens when a young, unhappy curly girl gets her first blowout or chemical straightening treatment: It can very quickly become an addiction. I know for certain I would've begged for a flat iron if they had been available at the time.

It seemed like no one around me—family, neighbors, or other kids—had crazy, curly hair, so to say I often felt left out and excluded by my brothers and sisters is an understatement. I also developed a massive inferiority complex (which I am glad to say I've overcome). Today, I don't mind standing out, but as a child, that's the last thing you want. I was bullied and teased mercilessly for my big, knotty, curly hair, from my first day of school until my last weeks of high school. When I sat in front of other kids, they would tell me to move because they couldn't see the

blackboard through my curls, or they would shoot spitballs at my hair along with other things that I found embedded in it at the end of the day. Because of this, I played truant a lot and got into trouble as a result.

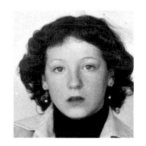

Dazed and uncurled, 13 years old

It's hard enough trying to fit into your immediate environment as a child, but it's even worse having hair that requires its own attention, like a constantly crying baby wanting to be fed. I often felt down and very sad. When I turned thirteen years old, I'd had enough of the constant taunting and bullying.

"I want to kill myself," I told my friend Dawn Hanley.

"Then can I have those earrings?" she replied. *What? No!* That snapped me

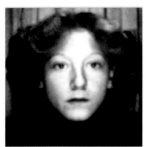

Sleepless from big rollers,
14 years old

out of it. (I call that the Dawn Hanley Effect.) I knew I wasn't going to end my life, but I was still miserable about my hair and myself, and all the negative references to it hurt deeply.

As I got older, I'd spend hours and hours trying whatever I could to make my hair flat and frizz-free. Before bed each night, I'd say a silent prayer that my curls would be gone for good in the morning and replaced with

> **Curls tend to take much longer to grow, so curlies often get frustrated when we hear, "It's only hair. It will grow!"**

the Farrah Fawcett hairstyle, which was straight hair that was feathered out on the side. When I realized this could happen only in my dreams, I tried tightly winding my hair around spiky bristle rollers and sleeping with them. None of this was realistic, but the pursuit of smooth strands was more important than sleeping comfortably. On rainy days, I would sneak out of school during lunch to go home and try to suffocate my hair under a ski mask for as long as I could. The results of all these efforts lasted for only minutes—especially because it is always drizzling in England! In retrospect, this obsession was similar to that of an addict: It consumed my every waking moment. Humid days could send me into a tailspin when, despite all my effort, my hair would frizz. I swear I could actually hear it crinkling upward and out.

HOW CURL BY CURL™ AND THE CG METHOD BEGAN

People often ask me when I decided to finally embrace my curls, but the truth is this: *I didn't decide. My curls decided for* me. When I was sixteen, I had a haircut that left my hair shorter on one side than the other. Some sections contracted back, and the rest projected outward or downward. (Yes, it looked as bad as it sounds.) When the stylist finished, I asked why my hair was totally uneven.

"It's even when it's wet," he said, pulling my strands downward to try to prove it. *But I don't wear my hair wet,* I thought. I was devastated, even more so when my boyfriend broke up with me right after he saw my haircut. I didn't blame him; I wanted to break up with me too! I had finally reached a curly lock bottom. I was done. I was tired of the stress, time, and relentless effort it took to control something that didn't want to be controlled. My hair decided it was time for me to give up fighting its nature.

Like planting a seed in a garden, I did nothing but patiently watch its curl pattern and shape emerge naturally and cleansed it with conditioner only. This eventually became the heart of the CG Method. Slowly but surely, I started to understand and respect my curls. I took a good, hard look at their shape and how each strand grew out of my head. I began to see them as part of nature, *my* nature, and learned to respect and accept the uncertainty of a day in the life of a curl. Like most curls, mine have a mind of their own. I never have the same hair two days in a row. It took years to learn to accept this and have realistic expectations. Over time, I began to appreciate my hair's whimsical nature and welcomed whatever dance it gave me. My mantra now is "What have you got for me today?" I can honestly say that my curls made me comfortable with surprises and raised my awareness of the natural world around us.

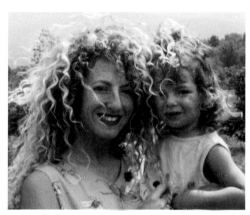

Happy days with Shey, my curly girl

Over months and years, and through lots of trial and error, I learned which products and techniques worked for my hair and which didn't. I stopped smothering it with sudsy, sulfate-filled shampoo with its salty lather that left my hair even thirstier, causing it to be brittle with knots and frizz. When I was in my twenties, I began what I call "co-washing," which is when you use silicone- and sulfate-free conditioner to cleanse your hair. Combined with the friction created by rubbing your scalp with your fingers, co-washing removes sebum, debris, and product residue without drying your hair or scalp. It may take some getting used to, since most of us have been brainwashed to believe that sudsy lather equals cleaner hair, but trust me, co-washing will leave your scalp and hair clean, healthy, and soft. Although I had never been happier with my curls and received many compliments,

I kept my co-washing ideas to myself. At that point, I was a hairdresser. How could I explain not using shampoo? To make matters worse, the blow-fry epidemic was in full swing. I admit my clients were a part of that—by my own hands!—but I was miserable doing so.

I also stopped cutting my hair for a couple of years, because it was only through length that I could understand the trajectory of my spirals. If we stop interfering, nature has a way of organizing itself. When I *did* trim my curls, I did so curl by curl, and while they were dry. After all, we wear our hair dry, so why in the world would we cut it when it's wet? Especially because curly hair is several inches longer when it's wet. Instead, cutting curls in their natural resting state lets you see their intrinsic shapes and forms.

At the time, my very loyal clientele had me cut their hair and blow it out. It was only after I'd gained their trust that they asked about my spirals and corkscrews and I began to share what I was doing: no shampoo, cutting dry hair curl by curl, and not touching my hair as it was air-drying. In truth, I never expected anyone to be interested—even when I was encouraged by David Schiller, a curly guy client who worked in publishing, to write a book about the techniques I had been using with curly clients for years at that point. Fast-forward to today, and I am certainly glad I did share my curl knowledge in the book *Curly Girl*, first published in 2002 and since revised and updated. I've also used what I've learned to create products that reinforce, preserve, and enhance your curl forms and personalities, not hurt them. I live in awe that my curls, which were once the bane of my existence, have become the vein of it, and I celebrate this regularly with millions of curlies around the globe.

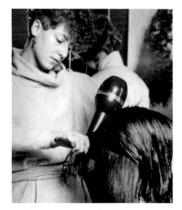

My face says how I feel about this activity!

Curly Kid Inspiration

Lindsay Wilson

During my son Daniel's first bath, I was terrified when I saw curls on his head. *Oh no! I have no clue about my own curls, and now my son has them too! We are doomed!* I thought. But then when my son was a toddler, I was voicing my frustrations to a curly-haired friend and she told me that I should see a dry curly cutter in the city for my own hair. I made the appointment immediately. The stylist recommended the CG Method. I went home and did all the research that I could about co-washing, joined a few support groups on Facebook, and ordered a copy of *Curly Girl: The Handbook.* My life was changed forever!

My hair began to bloom, like hydrated flowers in a field. I discovered a genuine love for my curls that is more than hair deep and discovered an incredible sense of self-confidence and being comfortable in my own skin. As I walked the journey with my own curls, I did the same with my son's. He was only a toddler, but I wanted to start him as early as possible, to avoid the same issues I had growing up.

Washing his hair with traditional shampoos used to be a nightmare, because the detergents in them always got into his eyes, which led to tears, as did detangling his hair. Shower times were something my son absolutely hated. Co-washing changed this very quickly! There were no more tears from detergents, and detangling was easier because his curls became very healthy. Now my son's curly hair routine is something that he enjoys, and we keep it very simple. A light, botanical, and silicone-free conditioner with lots of water and a bit of gel. Nothing else. He's only four years old, but sometimes he likes to apply the gel all by himself in front of the mirror.

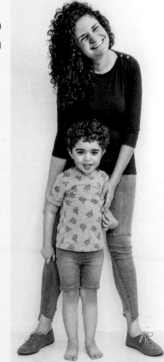

I created "Curly Girls Australia," the largest Facebook support group for curly hair in the country, designed specifically to teach the CG Method.

WHY *CURLY KIDS* NOW?

There are several reasons besides the fact that I have had the pleasure of meeting a lot of amazing people over the years, in person and on social media, who have requested a kids' book. First, curls are now more accepted as a hair type, but that doesn't mean parents or guardians always know how to care for them. This is especially the case if one or both parents has naturally straight hair and their child has curls. This scenario is more common than ever since the number of Americans married or in a partnership with a person of a different race or ethnicity has increased dramatically. As a result, chances are high that their children will have their own unique, beautifully mixed hair strands that are very different from their

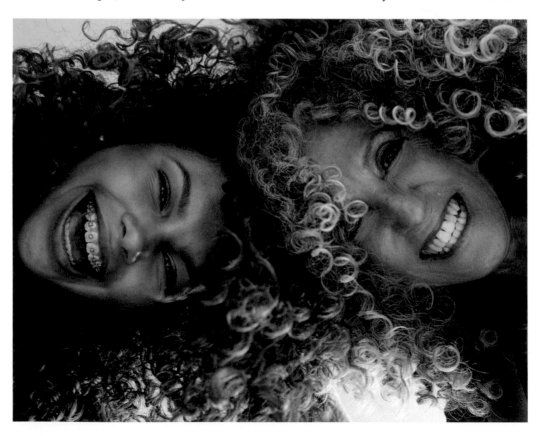

parents'. A perfect example of this is Kim Kardashian. On an episode of her reality show, Kim lamented her inability to style her then three-year-old daughter's very curly hair. Her child's beautiful locks are thanks to her father, Kanye West, and something Kim, with thick, blown-straight hair, didn't know how to handle. Kim Kardashian has time, resources, and experts to call on, so if *she* still needed help figuring it out, chances are many other parents do too.

International and multicultural adoptions are also important to mention because often parents adopt children of different races who have hair that's nothing like their own. Mark and Ann (not their real names) are a perfect example. They adopted their youngest daughter, Lea, from Ethiopia. Although their two biological daughters could run and play with their straight hair down, they soon learned that Lea's hair got intricately tangled if she did the same. Whereas their biological daughters' hair looked fine if it was washed daily, Lea's behaved better when it wasn't. I also met a Caucasian woman named Julie who adopted two African American children. She told me what she had overheard at church about her kids: "You can tell which children are adopted because their hair looks unkempt."

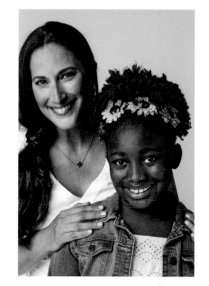

Another motivation for writing this book is the rising popularity of blowout bars, which are full of curly and wavy girls of all ages getting their temporary straightening fix. Often, moms who regularly straighten their own hair bring their daughters for blowouts. They have forgotten their curly hair (often willingly), and some actually believe that they do not have curls anymore. I can't tell you how many women I've heard say, "I used to have curls!" If you are born with curls, you will likely always have curls, no matter how much you try to heat-style them away. If you don't work with your

Curly Kid Inspiration

Kelly Skillestad

My son Connor's curls are a labor of love. There is a good eight-to-ten-inch spring to them. Luckily, he is a very patient, mature child who has accepted the work involved in keeping up with his curls. In the morning we must leave by 6:45, requiring him to rise quite early for his hair to be done. We plan wash days and refresh days very strategically, based on our busy schedule. If he goes too long between washes, the hair—especially in the back—gets tangled and matted from his car seat, pillows, sports helmets, gymnastics tumbling, amazing dance moves, pretend-play dress-up costumes, and so many people wanting to touch it.

Connor loves his curls and has never wanted his hair to be different, yet he has experienced kids being less than kind. We've worked through him being called

names like "golden noodle" and comments like "Your hair makes me hungry for noodles.

Connor's corkscrew curls

I'm going to eat your hair." Also, he's often mistaken for a girl, but he isn't bothered by it. An elderly woman at the grocery store expressed her amazement at the fact that it was his natural hair. Then she remarked, "You know, you should really straighten it. He would look . . . well, I probably shouldn't say it. But he would look less—" I told her to have a nice evening and then walked away. My guess is she was not a fan of interracial children and was attempting to tell me he would appear less African American if he didn't have the curly fro. But we love the fro. We celebrate Fro-Day when his hair gets super big! Connor has also come to love the "man bun," especially for soccer or swimming. It keeps the top curls from dangling in his eyes.

We have *loved* Connor's curls from the beginning. In fact, I set aside my own flat iron four years ago so that I could fully embrace his curl journey, and I have learned so much. His curls have fostered confidence! His unique curly hair has also given me the opportunity to teach him manners and gratitude for the compliments he gets.

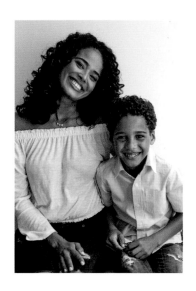

own hair you can temporarily lose your connection to it. That can result in confusion over what to do with your child's hair.

I've spoken to many women who tell me they stopped straightening their curls and returned to their hair's natural texture when their kids said, "Mommy, I want my hair to be like yours." I love that they want to be better hair role models for their kids! Now they need to be curl-*care* role models too. Although some women take motherhood as a time to embrace their curls, others are in such denial that they allow their kids as young as three years old to get regular blowouts. Many of my multitextural clients have said that having their hair chemically relaxed at a young age—three or four years old—was a rite of passage. Several years ago, actor Halle Berry took her ex-husband to court because he allegedly straightened their young daughter's hair. Good for her, because not only do those chemicals and tools damage the hair, but also straightening sent the message to their daughter that her natural hair was not good enough.

Another reason we wrote *Curly Kids* is more practical. With social media and the internet, there is more information than ever. Some of this advice and sharing is wonderful. However, all the insight, products, and techniques can be daunting as well as misleading and incorrect. *Curly Kids* can help clarify this information and bring curl care back to basics and simplicity because the truth is this: Your child's curls do need their own TLC, but it doesn't have to be difficult or complicated. In fact, when it comes to curls, less fuss will lead to better results.

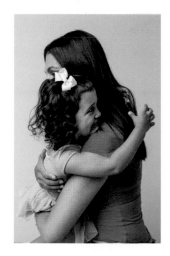

CURLS AND COILS ARE NOT A TREND. THEY ARE A LIFESTYLE.

In *Curly Kids*, we'll discuss caring for kids' hair at each age and stage—from infancy to young adult—and the nuances of each one. We'll focus on the various textures and how hair changes over the years, and share product insight and hairstyles. We'll help you handle curly hair dilemmas like lice, sports, and bedtime curls. One of the most important parts of this book is that we talk about cultivating a positive self-image—not always easy when your hair is viewed as something to hide or cover up—and what you can do to help your tweens and teens accept their hair.

Growing up, I longed for someone to help me understand why my hair did what it did. Actually, I used to dream about a fairy curl mother who would stop me on the street and say, "Listen. I know exactly what to do with your hair." Of course, it never happened, which is exactly why I've always wanted to be a curly mentor to others. And now it's your turn. Because if you picked up this book, clearly you

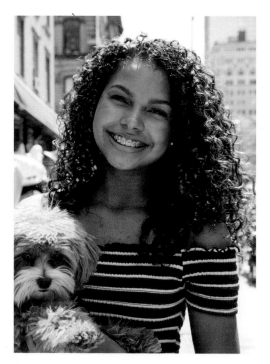

want to be an inspiration to the curly girls and boys around you. If *your* hair is curly, understanding your own curls better will help your child love his or her own. Just imagine being the curly girl or boy that *you* wished you had met as a child. Well, you are on your way! If your hair is straight, you may find your little one's curls hard to understand—both physically and emotionally. You picked up the right book. We're here to help.

Curly Kids is a book about loving the hair you were born with, but this is just a metaphor for loving all that we are and all that we have from a young age. And what could be better than that?

Curly Kid Inspiration

Glenis Santana

As a kid and teenager, I loved my curls wild and free and never liked to comb them. But my parents liked them only when they were straightened or put up neatly with tons of Alberto VO5. My mom would detangle my hair with a fine-tooth comb, which would take forever and cause a lot of tears, then she'd apply coconut oil and blow-dry it straight. When I got older, she would take me to a Dominican salon to have it blown out or set in rollers, which could take two to four hours.

When my son, Isaiah, was about eight months old, I saw the slightest wave at the tip of his crown and was so excited. By the time he was a year old, he had a head full of big, soft curls that became a little tighter as time went on. Today, he is six years old and we both absolutely love his curly hair. In fact, he made me promise that I will never make him cut it short.

In 2008, I received a diagnosis of severe chronic asthma. I was in and out of the hospital for long periods of time, and the medications made my hair brittle and dry, causing it to fall out. Because of this and not being able to take care

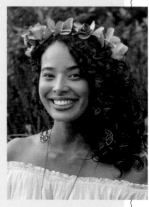

of myself, I had my hair straightened to make it more manageable. Eventually, my curls were replaced with a very light wave. I was so unhappy about this that I started looking on YouTube for tips, product suggestions, and information on curly haircuts. I vowed to never mistreat my hair again. Six months later, I was thrilled to celebrate one spiral curl. My husband thought I was crazy, but I knew life was coming back to me. After all, if your hair looks great, you feel great. Shortly after that, I had my first cut at Jersey Curl Salon with Rebecca, and I was in love. Thanks to the education process, the products, and the technique, my hair looks amazing. If it had not been for my condition and all that followed, I would have continued occasionally straightening my hair and using any kind of shampoo and conditioner. I know now that it takes time and dedication to show love to your hair—just like to any other part of your body—so it can love you back. I try very hard to pass this on to my kids and to teach them to embrace what God has blessed them with.

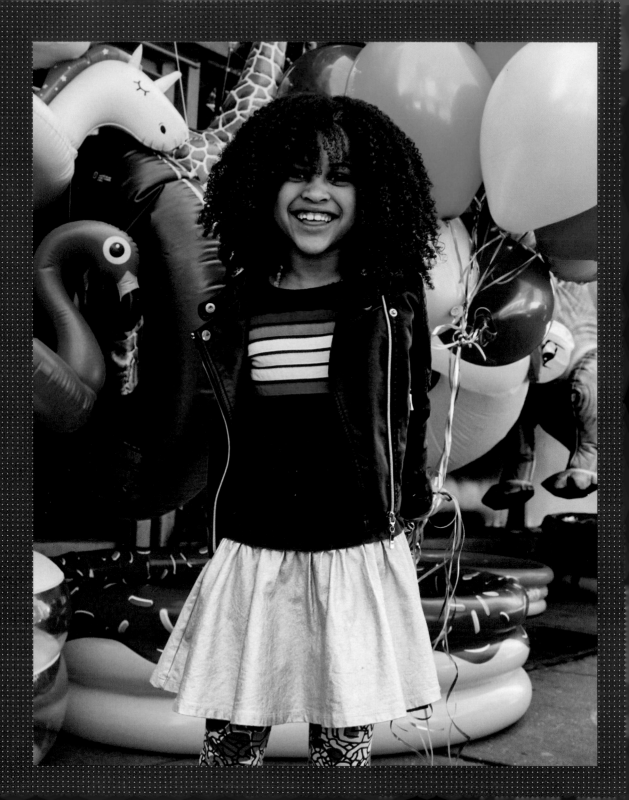

One

The Nature of Curly Hair & Care Basics

The art of looking after your child's curls is often more about what you *don't* do than what you do.

~~~~~~~~~~~~~

Our mission with this book is to connect you and your children to the hair that they were born with and to help you gain a mastery and understanding of the naturally curly ecosystem living on top of their heads (and maybe to think differently about your own). To care for it in the best way possible, it helps to understand a bit about the nature and science behind why curly hair does what it does. *It's a curly world after all.*

Although it's not always visible, hair appears on almost every surface of the human body except for the eyes, lips, palms of the hands, and soles of the feet. Infants are covered in what's called lanugo, the first hair to be produced by our bodies while we are still in the womb. Super-fine, soft, and unpigmented, it covers parts of the body and then disappears either by the time you are born or shortly thereafter. It is then replaced by vellus hairs—fine, wispy hairs that cover most of the body in areas that appear hairless, like your earlobes, nose, and forehead, among others. Often referred to as peach fuzz, these translucent hairs appear in larger numbers on children than on adults. They help sweat evaporate and regulate your body temperature. Curly hairlines can often remain "peachy" for life—another reason to be gentle on curls.

Hair on your head develops under your scalp, in a tiny sac called the follicle, which lies within the top two layers of the skin, the dermis and epidermis. When I think of one hair follicle, I envision it as a beautiful flower stem placed inside a narrow vase of water. The papilla of the hair follicle is an indentation at the bottom that feeds nutrients and oxygen to the hair through the blood vessels it contains. It is believed to be one of the most important structures related to the hair, because if it's damaged through illness or lack of nutrients, the blood supply to the hair will be negatively affected.

When the hair pushes up through the skin, it hardens and becomes the strand you see on your head. From inside, it will keep growing, lengthening the hair you see for three to five years, at a rate of about a half inch per month. Typically, it grows more quickly in the summer than the winter. Curlies often complain that their hair grows more slowly, but it just appears that way because its growth trajectory is a curved pattern rather than straight down. That said, we all have different growth rates. That is why even if you never cut your hair, it wouldn't just grow endlessly and hit the floor. We lose an estimated one hundred hairs a day. That may sound like a lot, but scientists say you have at least a hundred thousand hairs on your head at any given time.

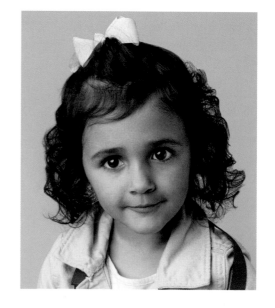

THE CUTICLE IS CRITICAL

If you examine a cross section of one strand of hair under a microscope, you'll see three centric cylinders similar to what you'd see in a cross section of wood. On the outside are tiny scales, which cover the cortex or center of the hair like tiles on a roof. Those overlapping "tiles" are called the cuticle and are essential to protecting each strand. When the tiles lie flat, they reflect light and your hair shines. When they're ruffled from outside interferences such as overtouching your hair with your hands, wind, harsh sulfates in shampoos, rubbing it with traditional terry-cloth towels, or using heat tools, chemicals, and brushes, your hair doesn't shine, because the surface isn't smooth. These things also damage hair by making the cuticle rough and scaly, so instead of lying flat, pieces of cuticle stick out and lock together like Velcro, causing knots, snarls, and tangles. The weather also affects the scales' ability to lie flat. In cold, dry weather they tend to be smoother than when the weather is warm and humid, because the moisture in the air makes the hair swell up.

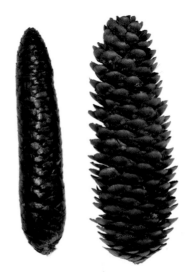

The cuticle resembles a pine cone. Smooth = moist cuticle. Open = dry, frizzed cuticle.

WHY CURLY HAIR IS DRIER

The hair is an appendage that grows out of the skin and is made up mainly of a protein called keratin that takes on a fiberlike consistency. This fiber must be thought of and treated like a priceless piece of clothing. After all, if we are lucky, we will wear this fiber on top of our heads every day of our lives. The goal should be to preserve and organize it and keep it healthy from the start. Each follicle that produces the hair on our heads is also home to sebaceous glands, which release

> "Eventually I knew precisely what hair wanted: it wanted to grow to be itself, to attract lint, if that was its destiny, but to be left alone by anyone, including me, who did not love it as it was."
>
> —ALICE WALKER

sebum, an oily substance that lubricates the hair. In curly hair, the shape and tightness of the follicle opening—where the hair is pushed through the skin on the scalp—has less room to produce sebum. That is one reason curly strands may be drier than straight.

Have you ever been told that brushing your hair a hundred times a night will make it shiny by dispersing the natural oil? Well, this is an old wives' tale. No one, especially curlies, has enough sebum to condition an entire head of hair. (If you do, then you may have a skin condition.) I was glad to learn that this is a myth, because a few times in my early life, I did try to brush my curls, hoping I'd get the oils to gush through to my ends. If you're a curly girl or guy, you know that the results were the opposite, making the hair frayed, frizzy, sparse, and even drier than before. Curlies need to use conditioners with extra moisturizing properties. But much more on that later!

DAM"AGE" TO HAIR

When the hair follicles are overexposed to things like chemicals for straightening and coloring, sulfate- and silicone-filled products, heat styling, and excessive tugging, it becomes impossible for the hair fiber to renew itself. A person may be young, but damaged hair can appear to be much older. Think of it like this: If you were to wear the same dress every day of your life, washing it daily with harsh detergents and dyeing, ironing, and exposing it to lots of friction and pulling, it would begin to deteriorate and definitely not look its best. The same goes for your hair. Unfortunately, many large hair-industry manufacturers promise us that their lotions and potions will repair this damage, which makes it okay to keep doing what you are doing without any consequences, right? Wrong.

Products that claim to repair all the damage to your hair in one shot are simply Band-Aids. They just disguise it temporarily. I know this is an inconvenient truth for those who want to continue to blow-fry and flat-iron their delicate hair fibers. But just as you can't unfry a steak, you can't unfry burned, damaged hair. Again, I urge you to be aware of products and oils that claim to restore, remedy, and repair the hair bonds. They are usually made up of silicone or resins that act sort of like superglue. Initially, they laminate the hair, which flattens the cuticle. This temporarily improves its appearance, but the key word here is *temporary*, and it's not sustainable. Over time, these products just entomb and suffocate the hair strands, because the cuticles are stuck and sealed together so tightly that nothing gets in and nothing comes out. The hair cannot breathe. This starves the hair of oxygen and makes it unable to receive true moisture from the atmosphere or from conditioner. This is a big problem, since hydration allows most things in nature to survive and thrive—including your hair.

> You are lucky to have every curl on your head—and they are lucky to have you.

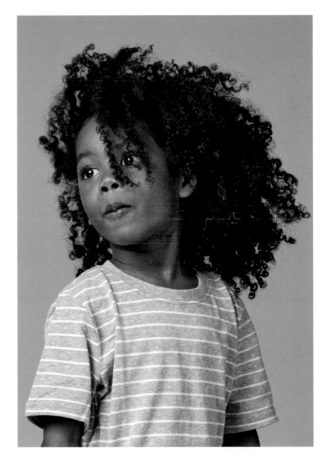

IT'S IN THE GENES

Genetics determines whether your hair is naturally curly, wavy, or straight, and the thickness of each individual strand. If you looked at a cross section of a very straight strand of hair under a microscope, you'd see that its shape is round. Think of toothpaste coming out of a tube. In contrast, a strand of curly hair looks elliptical, with a slight curve in the middle—like ribbon candy. The center indentation makes it flex and spiral—in other words, curl. Wavy hair, in contrast, looks oval under a microscope. Its spiral trajectory is looser, and it bends very slightly. Although hair can be chemically straightened or heat-styled, all forced applications are only temporary and unsustainable. You can't permanently change the shape of your hair, because you cannot change the structure of your follicles. They are predetermined by your DNA months before they are pushed out into the world from within the dermis. Although curly hair looks thick, the hair strands are typically very delicate and baby fine. Because of its acute reaction to atmospheric conditions thanks to its low moisture content, its expanding, spherical nature is an optical illusion, making it look like there is more hair than there is.

> **We *all* have good curls! How you handle and care for them makes the difference.**

FRIZZ EDUCATION

Often when curly girls and guys compliment my hair, they say, "*Your* hair is gorgeous, but I have bad curls." We *all* have good curls! How you handle and care for them makes the difference. One of the things that makes us unhappy with our hair is the CG nemesis: frizz. I prefer to call it a halo. Many women don't even know they have gorgeous curls, because their hair is suffocating under layers of dry frizz. I have become what I call a "frizzassist," so I can help you understand the science behind it.

Most of us spend days, months, and years scrubbing our already-dry hair with harsh, detergent-filled shampoos. Dehydrated from this rigorous cleansing process as well as from blow-frying, flat-ironing, and chemical treatments, the hair has to try to grab moisture from the atmosphere to survive. Thanks to their low molecular weight, little strands of your hair are literally swelling and lifting up off your head and quenching their thirst by absorbing the moisture from the water molecules in the air surrounding them. As a result, these lifted hair fibers create a poof that we call frizz. That is why curlies who straighten their hair don't like it when it rains or there's any kind of humidity. After being stripped from shampooing, parched from blow-frying, and singed from flat-ironing, every dry strand of hair is heading out as far as it can to get even a tiny drop of water. (I actually have a chart from the 1500s that uses hair as a weather barometer! It sounds crazy, but it makes sense.) However, there is a solution, and it's simple: moisture. Once the hair fibers are

Frizz is not a hair type. It's a head of curls asking for conditioner.

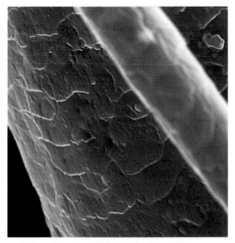

A strand of healthy, well-conditioned hair: The tile-like cuticle lies flat.

treated to a hydrating conditioner, they will hold on to the moisture that they need, and the dryness, volume, and frizz will go away. Curly hair is generally considered porous, but conditioner and its properties should help fill the holes, a bit like spackle on walls, and smooth the surface of the cuticle, giving it a little light reflection. Thanks to gravity, the weight of the conditioner also pulls the hair down and makes it appear longer in some cases. With consistent care and hydration, anyone and everyone can have beautifully defined curls without the frizz!

CARE BASICS FOR CURLY KIDS OF ALL AGES

CLEANSING, AKA CO-WASHING 101

Co-washing is the term I coined for "conditioning washing." It's also called the "no-shampoo" method and simply means that you're cleansing your hair with silicone- or sulfate-free conditioner rather than harsh, sulfate-filled (aka salt-filled) shampoos. However, not all silicone- and sulfate-free conditioners are created equal. For example, if it says it's sulfate-free but there's a lather, even a mild one, it means there are hidden sulfates in the product. It may take trial and error to find the right conditioner, but over time, your child's hair will be your biggest guide. I discovered this technique when I was eighteen years old and had ventured off to Hong Kong. The city's high humidity left my hair looking bigger and harder to manage than ever. My new hairdresser friend, Barry, suggested that from time to time, I wash my hair only with conditioner. Barry had no idea that he had just given me the best advice of my life. Within weeks, my hair had changed completely. It was more manageable and less frizzy, and my curls were softer to the touch and more defined—and my hair still felt clean and fresh. Cleansing with conditioner gives the hair an extra boost of moisture, which is something curly hair needs. However, this was my dirty secret for years. Why? I was a traditionally trained hairstylist, and all regular salon appointments at the time included a good old-fashioned hair scrub, so it didn't cross my mind to tell anyone I wasn't shampooing my *own* hair. That was probably a good thing. After all, if avoiding shampoo raises eyebrows *today*, can you imagine if I had dared to share this more than thirty years ago?

You don't drink salt water when you're thirsty. So don't put salt-filled shampoo on your thirsty curls!

Advice from a Stylist

Wafaya Abdallah, Oasis Hair Salon in Rockville, MD

When I was a child in Egypt, the women in my family mostly wore head coverings, so I knew that hair was significant and carried a lot of symbolism. As a youngster, I always had my hair tied up in pigtails or a braid of sorts. We immigrated to the United States, to Charlotte, North Carolina, when I was five years old. The first question I was asked was "Are you black or white?" The question that always followed was "Is that your real hair?" Already, at the age of five, my hair was frizzy and big, and I didn't feel like I belonged. As I grew into a tween, Farrah Fawcett came on the scene and really made life difficult for my hair and me. I longed and prayed for her feathered look, which was impossible for my hair in the high humidity of the South. When I became a teen, Donna Summer was popular. God bless her, because this made curls more accepted. I was fine with my natural curls and tried to understand them, but my mother would not have it. Being an Egyptian woman, she was convinced that straight hair—"like silk," she'd say—was more beautiful. I don't blame her. I know now that she was influenced by the culture. At the time, Egypt was a British protectorate, and many African countries were colonized by the Europeans. European features were regarded as more beautiful than African ones. As a result, Egyptians were straightening their hair and making sure the sun didn't darken their skin. The lighter their skin and the straighter their hair, the more highly their beauty was regarded.

Today, as a hairstylist specializing in curly hair, I have the opportunity to help girls, in our local community and all over the globe, understand the power in their authenticity through their curls. In a collaborative effort, curl specialists are able to use curly hair as the medium to showcase each individual's strength in their cultural identity. When we can empower curly girls to embrace the beauty of their cultural identity, we empower women to embrace their strength in society.

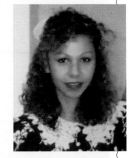

SOAPLESSLY DEVOTED TO YOU

This non-shampoo way of cleansing later became the basis for the Curly Girl/Curly Guy Method (also known as the CG Method) and various products that I created. Although banning sulfate-filled shampoo is a must for curly, wavy, or coily hair, which tends to be drier than naturally straight hair, doing so can benefit all hair types. At first you may miss seeing frothy, foamy lather when you co-wash your

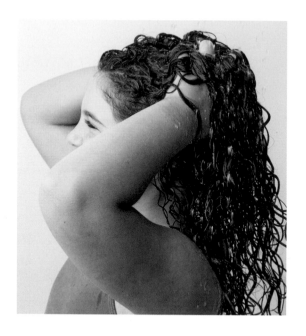

child's hair or your own. But trust me, lather doesn't do anything for hair fibers except cause dryness, tangles, and a matted feeling. Over time, these inorganic, sulfate-rich ingredients damage the hair and make it look and feel drier than ever. So please, give co-washing a whirl. Just know that old habits are hard to break! However, just as you get used to new foods and feeling different when you change your diet, you will begin to get used to a lack of lather, and the results will be worth it. Many people see the difference immediately. Although some people think it's shampoo and cleanser that clean hair, it's actually the friction of your hands that lifts away debris, dirt, and product buildup without removing your hair's natural oils. Taking a few days off between cleansings keeps your hair and scalp healthy by letting them breathe and prevents them from getting dried out.

SCIENCE FRICTION

Massaging the scalp gently but firmly with your finger pads not only cleanses the scalp, it also can help stimulate blood circulation, which can help ease tension and headaches and is believed to boost hair growth too.

CURL TYPES

Each person's curl type is determined by the shape of the follicle that the hair grows out of from the scalp. The flatter or more oval-shaped the follicle, the curlier the hair, while the more circular the cross section, the straighter the hair. Your child's curl pattern is also identified by the shape that the strands of hair make, whether they kink, curve, or wind around into spirals.

THE SPRING-BY-SPRING™ FACTOR

What I call the Spring-by-Spring factor is determined by measuring the distance between the length of a curl when it falls naturally and the length of a curl when it's fully extended. It's a way to determine which type of curl your child has. To measure the Spring-by-Spring factor:

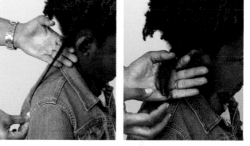

• Pull a fully dried curl downward to its furthest point and hold your finger where the strand ends.

• Leave your finger at the point where the strand ends while you let go of the curl.

• With a ruler, measure the distance between your finger and where the curl naturally ends. The number is your child's personal Spring-by-Spring factor.

9-to-16-inch spring = Fractal and Zigzag curls

9-to-12-inch spring = Corkscrew curls

5-to-10-inch spring = Corkicelli and Cherub curls

5-to-8-inch spring = Botticelli curls

2-to-4-inch spring = Wavy curls

About an inch = Light waves

FRACTAL CURLS

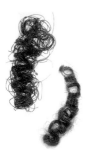

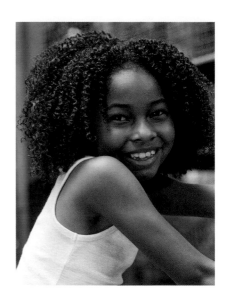

- Coily hair is commonly referred to as fractal curls, zigzags, or microcoils with natural volume.

- Strands form very tight, densely packed, self-similar curl shapes from zigzags to microcoil.

- These tightly packed coiled strands have a very tight zigzag pattern that is sometimes indiscernible when you look at the hair as a whole, but is apparent when you zoom in to each individual strand.

- Their circumference can be as small as the tip of a pen or as wide as an average knitting needle.

- The texture is naturally very dry to the touch and resembles beautiful moss cushions that you'd see in a forest bed.

- It can be soft and fine or wiry depending on how it is treated.

- Coils emerge directly from the scalp, and many are similar in shape throughout the head.

- They are prone to breakage from rough handling and harsh products.

- Coils don't change shape with the seasons.

- Co-washing should be done frequently to keep the texture hydrated and soft to the touch and to provide definition and buoyancy.

- To keep tighter coils freshly hydrated, you need to make sure no strand is left behind when you're generously infusing and applying conditioner.

- Try mixing styling gel and conditioner to create a cream gel. If absorbed correctly, it could add a little bit more moisture to co-wash-and-go styling. If it curdles, don't use it.

- Always apply your leave-in conditioner when hair is wet and saturated so you can achieve more definition without fused or frizzy strands.

- After air-drying, this hair type experiences the greatest amount of spring-back—about 75 percent or more. To temporarily lengthen hair, use a generous amount of leave-in conditioner, section the hair, and gently clip the bottom of each section with a hair clip to elongate the curls.

- Fractal textures are often naturally dry, so look for products without heavy oils or butters. These sit on the top of the hair, and as they build up, they create an impermeable barrier, blocking the hair from becoming saturated with water in the shower. This is very important, as the hair must be sufficiently soaked with water before cleansing and conditioning.

CORKSCREW CURLS

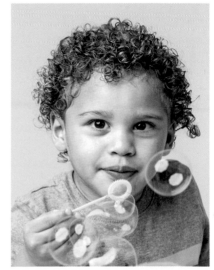

- These are tight corkscrew shapes that are about the circumference of a pencil.

- Strands are densely packed together, providing lots of natural volume.

- Hair appears thickly textured when you look at it all together but is actually baby fine and delicate if you separate the strands. This curl type is very delicate and can break easily.

- Corkscrews can soak up a lot of conditioner.

- This curl type has a high frizz factor if treated incorrectly.

- It tends to get tangled and snarled under the top layer of hair at the nape of the neck, caused by the natural movement of the head throughout the day, rubbing against clothes.

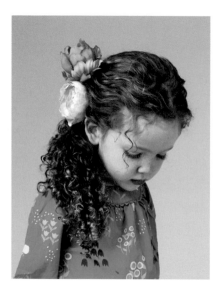

CORKICELLI

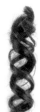

- Corkicelli curls are consecutive C's rotating and twisting into one another, and, with length, they ultimately create spiral curls.

- They are slightly larger than corkscrew curls but have similar characteristics.

CHERUB CURLS

- These are baby fine curl spirals that resemble the hair of a young child, whether you're eight years old or eighty.

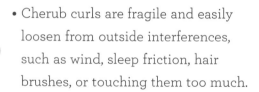

- Cherub curls are fragile and easily loosen from outside interferences, such as wind, sleep friction, hair brushes, or touching them too much.

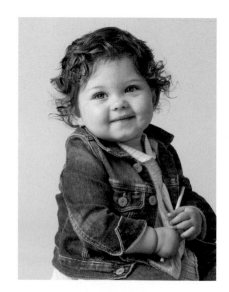

- They are almost weightless to the touch and have a translucency like a halo.

- They can be a variety of curl shapes, sizes, and lengths on one head.

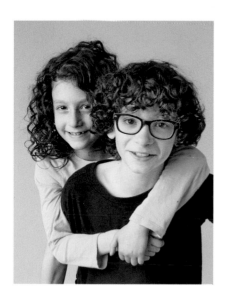

BOTTICELLI CURLS

- These are curls that vary in size and shape. Underneath you may have hermit curls that can shrink to half the length of those on the outside.

- Some curls tend to be looser, in the shape of soft S's, combined with those that are tighter.

- Curls are a fairly thick texture.

- The shape seems to wilt if it gets too long. This is because the weight of the top layer is bringing the hair down.

- Curls are looser during some seasons and tighter during others.

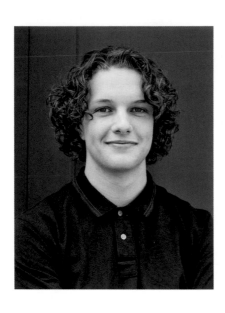

WAVY CURLS

- Wavy hair appears finer, tousled, but definitely not straight.

- Waves may not stay in the hair for more than a day.

- They can appear straighter if their shape is not encouraged and during the winter months.

- Waves seem to like products that give more hold, but too much of them can dry out the hair.

- Lighter styling potions and sprays work better than heavy ones that will weigh on each wave formation. Make sure you scrunch out most or all of the water before applying a leave-in conditioner or styling product.

- Wavy hair has little-to-no frizz factor and can have a natural shine if it is healthy.

LIGHT WAVES

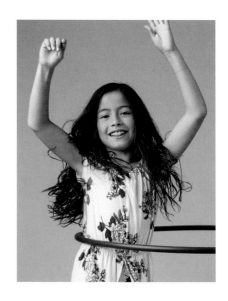

- These are natural surfer waves.

- Light waves can appear flatter at the crown with subtle S-shapes, which over time and with consistent care can become Botticelli curls.

- The wave starts from mid-length down.

- The waves are often thick, coarse, and more susceptible to frizzing if overly disturbed.

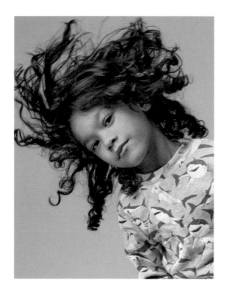

COMBO CURLS AND WAVES

- Waves may need some encouragement to reveal their shape, as gravity and too much product application can pull them down and stretch them out, making them appear straight. This is why some people don't recognize that they may have wavy hair.

- Hair may appear wavy after children come out of the shower and at the beach but may straighten out if the shape is not encouraged as it dries.

- Wavy hair may appear straighter in the winter.

- Wavy hair can range from baby fine and weightless to a coarser, thicker texture.

- Curls and waves can have a definitive S pattern or may stay flat and lie closer to the head.

- Children with wavy hair may have had straight hair when they were very young that became wavy after or around puberty. They tend to have an oily T-zone and scalp.

- Wavy hair can look flat and oily at the crown if touched too much.

- The ends of wavy hair can be dry if not hydrated correctly.

The CG Method

Although the details vary by age, and we'll talk about these differences in each age-specific chapter, there are some CG Method basics that apply to every curl type, from waves to corkscrews to super-tight fractal ringlets. You will be surprised at how simple they are and that it takes the same amount of time—or less—as a traditional cleansing routine. Every child is different, but many are ready to do their own hair around the age of nine or ten. All the better when you've started early and shown them the way.

- Wet your child's hair thoroughly. If it's too difficult to put your child's head under running bathwater, use a plastic cup, small pail, ladle, or toy watering can.

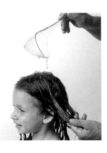

- Apply a silicone- and sulfate-free conditioner to the pads of your fingers on one hand and rub your hands together so it gets onto the pads of the other.

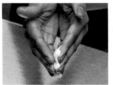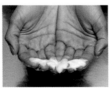

- The amount of conditioner you use depends on the length and thickness of your child's hair and takes some trial and error to determine. Generally, the tighter or drier the curl, the more conditioner you need to properly hydrate and detangle. Often, the amount used will change as your child's hair becomes healthier. For example, initially you may need to use more conditioner because the hair is so dry and thirsty; with time and consistent use, it will become healthier and more hydrated and will require less conditioner. Splay your fingers and place them directly on your child's scalp. Gently massage the scalp from the crown of the head to the nape of the neck. Be firm but gentle. Try not to over-whirl your child's hair around her head, because too much motion can cause frizz, knots, and tangles.

- Very gently let your fingers glide downward through small sections of your child's curls. This helps you carefully untangle knots, remove loose strands that have accumulated, and organize the curls into their natural position. Don't use a comb or brush.

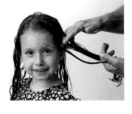

- Avoid forcefully pulling at knots and tangles. Instead, just apply more conditioner to those areas, with an added spritz of warm water to push the conditioner into the knot and detangle it more quickly.

- Rinse your child's hair with a plastic cup, pail, ladle, or watering can or by cupping your hands together and putting them under the running water. Deciding whether to 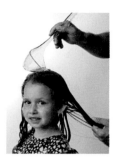 rinse out all the conditioner or just some of it also takes some trial and error as you see how the hair responds best. You can rinse out most or all of it if your child has looser curls or waves. For coarser, tighter curls, leave in more conditioner, because those curls tend to be drier and more frizz-prone. Some people with really tight curls may not need to rinse at all. I know that sounds unorthodox, especially since we're so conditioned (pun intended) to rinse thoroughly for fear that the hair will be weighed down or greasy. But in reality, curly hair *needs* that extra moisture to remain hydrated and frizz-free. (The word *greasy* is almost never part of a curly girl's or guy's vocabulary.) You may also worry that leaving conditioner in will make the hair crunchy, hard, and sticky, but that should not happen when you're using products that don't contain sulfates and silicone.

- *Squeeze-quench* is a term I use to describe the process of using your hands to squeeze small sections of your child's hair in an upward motion toward the scalp. You can have your child tilt his or her head to one side and then the other or have them bend over at the waist. If you hear a luscious squishy sound, that means your mission of hydration has been accomplished. When you squeeze-quench, a milky residue of excess water and conditioner may seep through your fingers. The hair naturally drinks up and absorbs the conditioner it needs to stay properly hydrated and usually drips and releases what it doesn't. Have a plastic container on hand to collect the milky residue. If you feel like the hair needs more conditioning, you can recycle it back into your child's hair and rinse again, or you can use it after they get out of the bath or shower as a leave-in for further hydration.

- A traditional terry-cloth towel has fibers that can ruffle the hair's cuticle, causing frizz and disturbing each curl's natural shape. 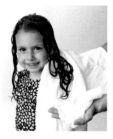 With a traditional towel, you also can't feel the water content in the hair and how much water you want to take out or keep in. This also applies to microfiber towels. So once your child is out of the bath or shower, use a paper towel, an old T-shirt,

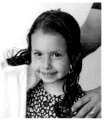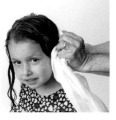

or multipurpose towels, which you can find at Home Depot or at office supply or other big-box stores, to gently squeeze small sections of the hair upward toward the scalp. This will remove excess water and encourage each curl's natural shape.

SOAK IT UP

Multipurpose paper towels can be reused. Just hang them to dry. When you use them again after your child's next co-wash, the conditioner in the paper towel will reactivate and hydrate the hair. Think of it like a conditioning towelette. Personally, I do this for weeks until the towel has had enough.

- Try not to touch your child's curls as they dry, and tell your child not to touch them either. Also be mindful when dressing your child, because pulling clothing on and off over the head can cause strands to disperse and frizz.

- Long or thick hair can take a while to dry, so if a bath or shower is part of your child's pre-bed routine and you don't want her going to sleep with wet hair, you can use a blow-dryer with a diffuser or a hooded helmet dryer (surprisingly inexpensive online).

- Try not to co-wash your child's hair every day. Over time you will figure out how often co-washing is necessary and how your child's hair is affected by weather, activities, and age. That said, in the beginning, when you're weaning your child (and possibly yourself) off shampoo, you may want to stay on your usual cleansing schedule but use a sulfate- and silicone-free conditioning product. You should very quickly see the hair becoming more hydrated and manageable.

- On bath and shower days when you are not planning to co-wash, put your child's hair up in a pineapple (see page 51) so it doesn't get wet. The humidity from the bath or shower may interact with the curls. If it becomes frizzy, just scrunch in some of Co-Wash in a Bottle (see the recipe on page 170).

- Curls can change daily—even hourly—because of outside influences like weather and hard or soft water. Simply adjust the amount of conditioner you use from one season to another, when you travel to a different locale, or when kids are going to summer camp or changing their activities.

- When you switch to the CG Method of co-washing, there may be an adjustment period, something I hear from CG Method newbies. Some see an immediate difference; for others, it takes a lot longer for the beauty of your child's curls to emerge. It all depends on application technique and the quality of the ingredients in the products as well as the length and thickness of the hair and the amount of damage the hair has endured.

- If you use styling gel on your child's damp hair—for special occasions, for instance—once the hair is dry, it may feel as if a light, sometimes stiff film of gel is surrounding each curl. Some people like to leave the hair in this "product cast" to preserve the hairstyle for later in the day or if it's raining. Other times, you may want to soften the look of your child's curls or you may not like the wet appearance of the product cast. In that case, once the hair is completely dry, simply scrunch small areas of the hair upward to dissolve the product cast. Then insert your fingers underneath the hair at one side of the nape of your child's neck. Have her tilt her head to that side while you gently shuffle your fingers at the roots to open the curls. Repeat on the other side of the head for a softer curl.

AERATE THE SOIL, AERATE THE SCALP

For extra root lift and to aerate, refresh, and open up your child's curls at any time, have her bend forward at the waist. Then place your hands lightly at the scalp near the crown of the head and gently shuffle the hair with the pads of your fingers. Remove your fingers carefully without raking them through the hair to avoid disrupting the curls. Have your child slowly bring her head to an upright position. Once she's standing, have her tilt her head back to look at the ceiling and gently shake the hair back and forth. This can be done on freshly co-washed hair or once it has completely dried.

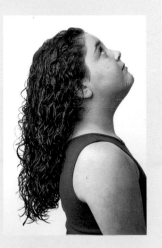

THE BEST WAY TO "COMB" CURLS

If you are looking to cultivate your child's curl formations, my comb of choice is always your hands, used when your child's hair is wet and protected by conditioner. Because your hands are a part of you, their touch is gentler and allows you to connect to what the hair may need. Brushes and combs don't have any sensory feeling toward your hair fiber. They disrupt the natural shape of each curl, coil, or wave and can fuse curls to one another so the definition of each curl is no longer visible. This can also cause frizz and affects the curls' memory because they are constantly being disturbed. Also, many people use a heavier hand with a brush or comb and use these tools when the hair is wet.

On dry hair, you can use an old-school hair pick, but only to very gently give the roots some aeration and lift. Lightly insert the pick at the roots at the base of the scalp and gently shuffle it upward. Then tilt the head and repeat on both sides of the parietal ridge (the curve of the head), gently lifting the hair there too. Remove the pick from the hair without raking it through the entire length of the curls.

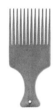

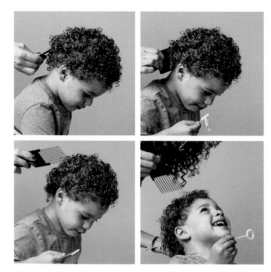

Gentle use of a hair pick give curls a lift.

That said, it would be unrealistic for me not to mention traditional brushes and combs. If you insist on using one or the other on your child, make sure both the hair and the brush's bristles are coated with conditioner beforehand. This creates something of a protective barrier as you pull the brush through your child's curls. Brushing the hair when it's unprotected opens the cuticle, creating a halo of frizz that attaches itself to the open cuticles on the neighboring strands of hair, causing knots. Try not to tug or rip through the hair, because these organic strands don't renew themselves when torn. Products that claim to repair hair in one shot don't work. Don't allow your child's hair to get worn-out and treated like an old cloth.

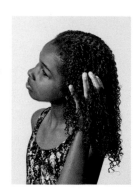

PRODUCTS—WHAT TO KNOW

It's important to read the ingredient lists on the labels of your products and teach your kids to do the same. **Make sure these ingredients are not in your products:**

SULFATES AND SODIUM. These are forms of salt. Sodium lauryl sulfate (the harshest), ammonium laureth sulfate (also harsh), and sodium laureth sulfate (harsh) are the most common. These substances are found in all lathering shampoos, body washes, toothpastes, and household cleaners. Yes, the same harsh ingredients can be in your shampoo *and* your toilet bowl cleaner! Often, they're used because they are an inexpensive way to create lather, which we've been led to believe is necessary for us to get clean. They are designed to get rid of oils in the hair and grease on dishes, but they harden and calcify the hair and quickly dehydrate it, along with the scalp. Curls are naturally drier than naturally straight strands, so sulfates or other dehydrating ingredients can lead to unhealthy hair. After all, you don't drink salt water to quench your thirst, so why would you use it to hydrate your hair? These ingredients are also universally known among chemists as skin, scalp, and eye irritants. It may say "sulfate-free" on the label, but check to make sure none of the ingredients listed above are in it. Again, soap lather, which comes from sulfates, does *not* cleanse the hair in the way you may think. It *dries out* the hair. Sulfates are a massive sham—as in "sham"poo. Sulfate-free means lather-free.

SILICONES, also known as polysiloxanes, are ingredients in sealants for cars, adhesives, lubricants, medicine, cooking utensils, and thermal and electrical insulation because they are typically heat resistant. Some common forms are silicone oil, silicone grease, silicone rubber, silicone resin, and silicone caulk. Their purpose is to repel heat, water, and light and form a watertight seal. That is fine for a roof, the outside of a car, and your shower, but these unnatural ingredients are bad for hair of any type. When you apply silicone to hair, it prevents moisture and oxygen from getting in. This suffocates each strand as it builds up. Depending on your level of awareness, you might not notice it for weeks or months. Although silicone-based hair products boast about the shine they leave behind, it's a plastic-like shine. It's fake and unsustainable. Over time, they leave hair looking dull,

Curly Kid Inspiration

Jillian Saez

As a preschooler, my son Mason was often mistaken for a girl. This made him very aware of his long hair—but he liked it anyway. Then he was bullied in kindergarten. When he would walk into the restroom, boys would yell, "Ewww, there's a girl in here. Cover yourself" or they'd push him out and tell him, "You can't be in here because you're a girl." It made him cry and want to cut his hair. But I wanted Mason to know that there is no rule about what boys' or girls' hair should look like and he is perfect just the way he is.

Luckily, we were able to stop the bullying, those kids were given consequences, and we kept Mason's hair long. A couple of months later, I decided to make him an Instagram page so that I could find inspirational curly guys and kids. At some point, I shared his story about being bullied, and the number of curly men who reached out to Mason with video messages and words of encouragement made him feel special and accepted. It also made him realize that he wasn't the only boy with long, curly, beautiful hair.

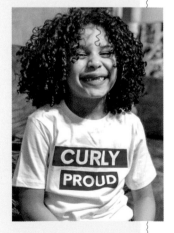

because the silicone sticks to the hair strands like glue and doesn't readily wash out. It's like getting a clear gum stuck in your hair. It may be removed *only* by being cut out. The film left behind may clog the skin and may cause hair loss. It is designed to repel water, preventing the hair from absorbing the moisture it needs. These also go by the name "anti-humectants." Beware. You especially don't want silicone in any styling products you or your children use. Since these are designed as leave-ins, the ingredients stay in the hair like a squatter who never wants to leave. They basically turn organic hair into synthetic, doll-like hair.

Unfortunately, you may not notice the effects of silicone buildup for weeks or months, and by the time you do, your hair will be fully coated. Silicone is even more damaging when intense heat is applied because it laminates the hair. Many products encourage this and call themselves "heat-protective" stylers or something similar. However, the last thing they do is protect. Instead, they encase the hair strands in a plastic-like, heat-resistant coating. This is part of the very pricey trademarked Brazilian blowout. The long-lasting effect is no joke; the hair is stuck until the silicone is cut out.

ALCOHOL. Curls should be seen and not heard, but alcohol in gels can cause hair sound effects. The right gel will leave your hair frizz free, bouncy, and touchable, and all you'll hear is how curl'ishious you look! Certain alcohols are okay if they're in your conditioner, gels, or cleansers—like cetyl alcohol. But other types, such as those used in gels, can be extremely drying and cause frizz. Plus, unlike sulfate-free cleansers, which are in the hair only a brief time and get rinsed out thoroughly, styling gel will stay in curly locks for a day or two or three or more. If it contains alcohol, it will spend those days sucking up your strands' moisture—like when you get to the bottom of your favorite drink and slurp it up with a straw—and preventing any new hydration from getting in.

PARABENS. Parabens are one of the most widely used preservatives added to cosmetics (as well as foods and drugs) to ward off the growth of bacteria. Those you'll typically find in the ingredient list are methylparaben, propylparaben, and butylparaben. In recent years, they've become controversial as experts question whether they are safe. Some say they may be linked to cancer. Despite the health issues, many chemists still believe parabens are the best preservatives ever.

FORMALDEHYDE may be the scariest ingredient on the list of no-no's. It is a known human carcinogen, and research on animals suggests it can be absorbed through the skin. Manufacturers often add it directly to products as a preservative, but it can also be released over time from other types of preservatives through a chemical process. The formaldehyde releasers have different names, and it's not always clear what they actually are. In 2013, hundreds of American women sued Unilever after experiencing hair loss, burned scalps, and broken or discolored hair after using an at-home hair-smoothing product. The product contained a formaldehyde-releasing ingredient. Formaldehyde can also be found in some chemical hair-straightening treatments and is often activated through heat. In some cases, stylists wear industrial-strength masks while doing these treatments. I think that's cause for concern. Stylists who have applied these treatments have complained of nosebleeds, throat and eye irritation, and difficulty breathing. In studies, researchers have even found significant levels of formaldehyde in products labeled "formaldehyde-free." Other dangerous chemicals like methanol and ethanol were also found. Despite this, formaldehyde is legal in personal-care products in the United States, unlike in the European Union, which has restricted its use, and in Sweden and Japan, where it's banned completely from cosmetics and toiletries.

ALSO AVOID

• Triclosan, a highly toxic antibacterial ingredient.

• Artificial fragrances, which studies have shown can even migrate into breast milk.

- Phthalates (pronounced *thay-lates*), ethyl acetate, galaxolide, BHA, BHT, tolunene, and styrene. These can be toxic to humans, animals, and the environment.

FRIZZ IS JUST A CURL WAITING TO HAPPEN, AND A CURL IS FRIZZ WAITING TO HAPPEN

Although frizz has gotten a bad rap, it's not necessarily a bad thing. It has taken a lifetime for me to feel this way, but I personally like my halo at times and have clients who feel the same way. I think that if hair is healthy and the curls are basically well defined, a little frizz can be great for added volume.

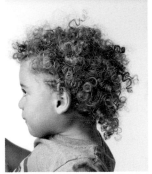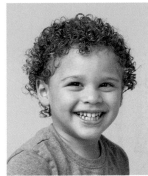

From frizz to fantastic

In fact, I often receive more compliments on days when I haven't fought the frizz! And if I'm having a bad curl day, I am the only one who seems to think it's bad. I have long accepted frizz as one of the ways in which my curls sometimes choose to express themselves or respond to the weather, and I have stopped taking it personally. This has given me a sense of freedom. However, if you're not ready to embrace your halo, here are some tips to eliminate it.

- On rainy or high-humidity days, wet hair thoroughly and use extra conditioner to seal the cuticle. It will help elongate the curls so that gravity directs them downward instead of out.

- Don't have your child linger too long in a steamy bathroom after showering and before preparing to style the hair. The humidity can open up the hair's cuticle, causing a higher frizz factor.

- Give curls a last cool rinse to seal the cuticles before styling. Fill a bowl with cool water, and if you're both really determined, put ice in it. Get a plastic cup or soup ladle and pour the water over your child's hair while they're still in the shower or bath and looking up at the ceiling.

- Once they're out of the bath or shower, have your child lean forward. With your hands or a paper towel, scrunch out as much water and conditioner as possible.

- Immediately scrunch in a gel. Knowing the amount you need takes some trial and error. Start with a small amount and add as needed. Distribute it evenly throughout the landscape of the hair, leaving no curl behind.

- Bring the head to an upright position and let your hands graze over the canopy of the hair in a downward motion to keep the cuticles smooth.

- Don't touch your child's hair once you've applied gel, no matter how tempted you are—or your child is—to pat even a single strand into place. That is a general rule for curlies, but it's particularly important on frizz-prone days.

- Keep the hair in a gel cast (meaning don't touch it, fluff it, or, especially, use any implement on it). If your child has a party, prom, or other extra-special occasion later in the day, the gel cast can protect his or her locks and encourage the curls to stay vacuum packed until you want them to open up to their natural state. Here is one way to apply a light coating of gel: After cleansing and styling, spritz spray gel onto a scarf and lay it loosely over your child's hair. Clip or tie the scarf at the nape of the neck for five to ten minutes. The scarf acts as an opposing weight that won't allow the cuticles on the canopy of the hair (the frizz) to rise.

- Once it's time for the party, you can open the gel cast by simply scrunching small sections of the hair upward (just like you do when squeeze-quenching). Do this either with your child standing bent over at the waist or with her head tilted to one side, then the other.

Advice from a Stylist

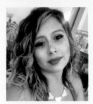

Veronica Tapia, owner of Jersey Curl Salon in Cliffside Park, NJ

My mom always kept my curly hair on the longer side, with no layers. Having my mom brush my hair with a really hard bristle brush was torture! Because we kept my hair long with no layers, I never knew I had wavy/curly hair until I was about thirteen years old. When I did discover it, I loved it. As I got older, I learned what I was doing wrong with my curls and changed my whole routine. It was actually easier to just leave my hair natural, and I felt prettier. I love taking care of kids' hair at the salon and helping parents understand how to handle their kids' hair.

- Today, there are many good products for curls, and curly specialists who know what they're doing with our hair. It's worth it to do the research and find them.

- Never use a brush or comb on curly hair!

- Read about the CG Method, from *Curly Girl: The Handbook.*

- Beware of false CG information on the internet. Check your sources or DM Lorraine on Instagram.

- Get a pair of high-quality cutting shears and cut your child's hair at every C. Little snips make a huge difference.

- Have your child's hair cut dry.

- Don't be afraid to try to condition and detangle your kids' hair. Many kids have little tantrums, and moms easily give up. Detangling and conditioning are like brushing your teeth and flossing: They're a must! And it gets easier as hair gets healthier.

- Moms at the salon always say how expensive good-quality curly hair products are—especially when they have more than one child. An average twelve-ounce bottle of conditioner could easily be used up after just two or three cleanses. I tell them to focus on getting just a good silicone-free conditioner and never to use shampoo.

- Gently braiding the hair while it's damp with leave-in conditioner helps keep the hair from tangling, especially if your child showers at night. Then you can just refresh the curls the next morning with a mix of water and conditioner, such as Co-Wash In a Bottle (see the recipe on page 170) and add some product.

CLIP IT, LIFT IT

A lot of curly girls and boys complain about their hair being flat at the roots. There are two ways to give this area some lift: One is by strategically using clips; the other is with two hair picks.

FOR ROOT LIFT WITH CLIPS

• Many curlies worry about placing the clips incorrectly, but I always tell them not to overthink this, because it's actually very simple. Place clips along the part at the spot on the curl where the roots meet the scalp. This helps preserve the curls' intrinsic pattern. If you place the clip away from the scalp or if it happens to dislodge, you're actually adding more weight, which pulls the hair downward, making it appear flatter. It can also expose gaps and cowlicks in the hair.

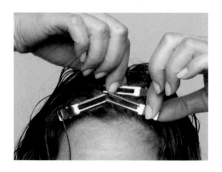

• Open the clip, slide it in at the base of the scalp, feel the lift at the root, and leave it. When you start to understand your child's hairscape, you'll see where the gaps and cowlicks reside (usually at the crown). This is the basic clip technique and usually requires two to three clips.

• The hair on the sides of the head at the point where the head curves and at the crown, typically where a cowlick would be, can look flat when it dries. As hair gets longer, this flat spot is more apparent. In that case, place one clip at the crown.

• You can use bobby pins instead of clips. Those that are the same color as the hair can be invisibly woven into the roots, and bobby pins are often easier to remove than clips.

• Once hair dries, use care to patiently remove the clips or bobby pins, because hair swells during the drying process and can wrap around the clip the way ivy wraps around a tree trunk. To take them out, it's important to use *both* hands. Hold the piece of hair gently with one hand, and then open the clip and slide it out with the other. This anchors the hair and ensures that you are not ripping the clip and any hair out.

GETTING LIFT WITH TWO PICKS

This method not only gives the roots some lift but also helps curls dry faster, because you're picking the wet hair up off the scalp, allowing it to aerate.

• Hold a pick in each hand slightly above the head with the pick teeth facing inward, toward each other.

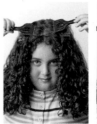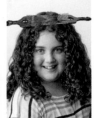

• Gently slide them into the hair at the side of the head at the crown until they meet and their teeth lock together. As you do so, you should feel the hair lift ever so slightly.

• Leave the picks in until the hair dries. Yes, it looks a bit strange, but it works, and when you take them out, it does not cause frayed hairs the way bobby pins or hair clips can.

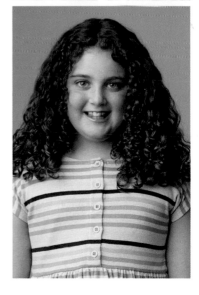

• Just like you need to be careful removing clips when the hair dries, be careful removing the picks, because the curls swell when they dry and may wrap around the teeth of the pick. Hold the hair lightly with one hand and gently pull one pick out with the other hand. Repeat on the other side.

• On dry hair, you can use the picks to refresh the scalp on second- or third-day hair and give it lift. Simply wet or spray the picks with the Mist in You Lavender All-Purpose Herbal Cleanser or apply Halo Goodbye Hair Gel and insert as described previously. See Chapter 6 for recipes for the mist and gel.

LIFT WITH HEADBANDS

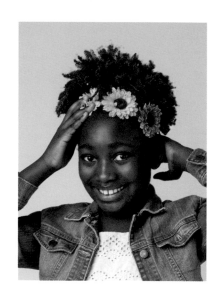

Another option for lift is a lightweight headband. (See page 170 for instructions on how to make your own.) This helps give the hair a little lift at the crown. It also gets the hair out of your child's face and stops her from touching her hair while it's wet. Simply put the loose-fitting headband around your child's neck and pull up gently, allowing the hair to be loosely held back from the face.

BEDTIME CURLS

When it comes to curls, sleep matters too. Tossing and turning can cause a lot of friction, which can ruffle the cuticle of the hair. This can cause frizz, knots, and frays, especially with long hair. Also, getting curls ready for bed the right way makes it easier to manage them in the morning. Preparing the hair properly helps if it rains in the middle of the night, because that change in the weather can have an effect on hair. (This also helps if your child is sick and spending a lot of the day in bed.)

Here's how . . .

• If possible, get your child a sateen or silk pillowcase. This reduces friction on the hair, which decreases frizz and split ends.

• **THE VEIL** hairstyle is a good option if your child has long hair. Have your child lie down and spread the hair over the pillow almost like you are spreading out a veil. If she can sleep on her back, a pillow tucked under the knees can be a very comfortable and ergonomic sleeping position. This is great for children who don't move a lot in their sleep.

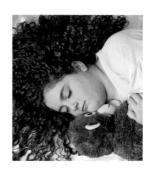

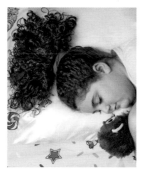

• **THE PINEAPPLE** may be more realistic for kids who move a lot in their sleep. Have your child bend forward at the waist and tilt the head forward. Gather the hair gently at the center of the top of the head with a fabric-covered ponytail holder, ribbon, or scarf. Loop the band around the hair two or three times and pull the hair all the way through. This prevents the ends of the hair and the curls at the nape of the neck from getting knotted and prevents frizz if it rains during the night.

• For a **LOOPED BUN**, have your child bend forward at the waist and tilt the head forward. Gather the hair at the crown using a fabric-covered ponytail holder. As you loop the band the second or third time, don't pull the hair through, so that it resembles a looped fan. This is good for thick or wavy hair.

In the morning, very gently remove the ponytail holder, ribbon, or scarf from the Looped Bun or Pineapple. Spritz your child's hair with lavender spray, or wet your hands slightly, place your fingertips lightly on her scalp, and shuffle the hair at the roots. Then let the hair settle. This will loosen curls without disfiguring them.

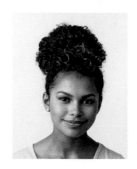

TALES OF PONYTAILS

Ponytails and childhood go hand in hand. But the key to healthy scalps and hair is starting kids off right with the proper pony technique from day one.

• Use fabric-covered ponytail holders. Most elastic bands—especially those with metal—can pinch, gnaw, and tear the hair. Some can also saw on the hair, causing damage when the head moves back and forth while your child is doing things like running and skipping.

• Make pony- and pigtails a little loose. Tight ponytails may seem like a good idea because they appear to secure the hair, keeping it out of your child's face. But a tight ponytail every day can pull on the hairline. This can cause something called traction alopecia, which is when the hairs fall out or become sparse, causing a receding hairline. In some cases, these hairs won't grow back. Too-tight ponytails can also cause headaches.

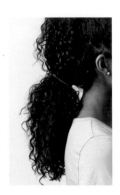

• If hair is thick, make sure it's not soaking wet when you put it in a ponytail for the rest of the day. This can cause mold and odor to set in. Let hair air-dry as long as possible or use a bonnet dryer or diffuser before *very* loosely tying it back.

WHY YOUR CHILD'S NATURAL HAIR IS BEST

Here are some great reasons for you to celebrate your kids' natural hair and teach them to do so too. Sharing these reasons with your child as early as possible will help make embracing her hair just a natural part of life.

- Your children's lives will not revolve around their hair, so they will be able to fully appreciate all activities and weather conditions. They will never skip a swim, workout, or run through a sprinkler because they're worried about their hair. Our hair is a part of us, not apart from us. It goes with us wherever we go, so why not love it?

- You're helping the environment. Avoiding sulfate-filled products means you're not washing these detergents into our waterways. Not using blow-dryers and flat irons saves electricity. You're also using less hair-care product and therefore not polluting our oceans with the packaging.

- With air temperatures warming up and more rain, it's harder to keep hair that's been blown straight or flat-ironed from curling up. If you don't flatten your hair, you won't have to worry about it un-flattening!

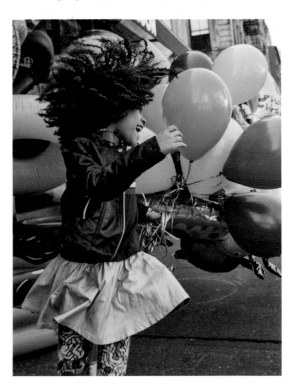

- Your children can travel light. No lugging loads of products and appliances.

- You'll save money on products, appliances, and salon appointments and can pass these savings on to your kids when they get older.

- Most important, loving their curls gives your kids a sense of confidence and freedom and teaches them to love being themselves. Priceless!

Curly Kid Inspiration

Ledia Andrawes

Growing up, I felt like my hair was the reason I was not accepted by the "cool" kids at primary school. So I thought my hair made me ugly and unwanted. I blamed it for so much. That is not even including the pain and drama of maintaining it. I dreaded wash day. It would take three hours to wash, condition, and detangle it, drench it in oil, and then put it in a plait. My mum would sit on a chair, and I would sit at her feet on the floor while she would sort it section by section and detangle it after I'd come out of the shower. It would hurt so much. It was a pain for her too, I could see. So when I was twelve years old and my mum suggested chemically straightening my hair, I was ecstatic! Finally, I could be like other girls. Finally, I could be freed from this hair trauma! I straightened it for a long time.

In the past few years, I decided to go naturally curly. I was living in Nairobi and saw that my hair and its texture could be perceived as beautiful. This gave me the courage to take the leap and go natural. However, it was more than just that. I had a realization that in my culture,

in my family, only straight, smooth, white-people-looking hair was beautiful. What "we" have is inferior, untamed, and unsightly. I grew tired of trying to fit into such a narrow version of beauty that was so exclusive. But not everyone felt this way.

We lost my grandmother recently. During the planning meeting with the funeral director and about fifteen members of my extended family, we discussed dress code. We would all wear white, not the usual black attire. This was to celebrate my grandmother and her life, not just mourn her departure.

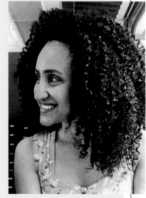

"Ledia, how are you going to wear your hair?" one family member asked.

"Maybe it would be better not to wear it like it is now for the funeral," said another.

"Hold on: What is wrong with her hair?" another asked. This discussion went on for a couple more minutes. I watched in amazement that my hair could be a topic of discussion in that setting, at that time. It clearly meant something: Maybe it would reflect badly on the family if I didn't have my hair in order. They did not mean to be controversial; it came from a deeply embedded belief that being beautiful meant having your hair tamed.

Everywhere, from supermarket checkouts to airport security, people tell me how much they love my hair. I now see my hair differently than I once did: It is absolutely fabulous in its own big and curly way.

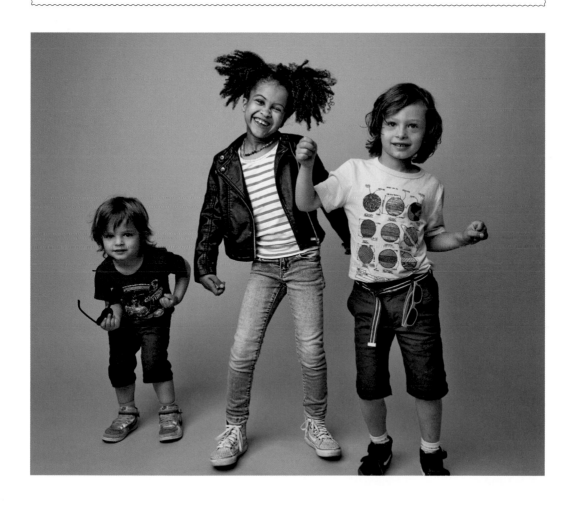

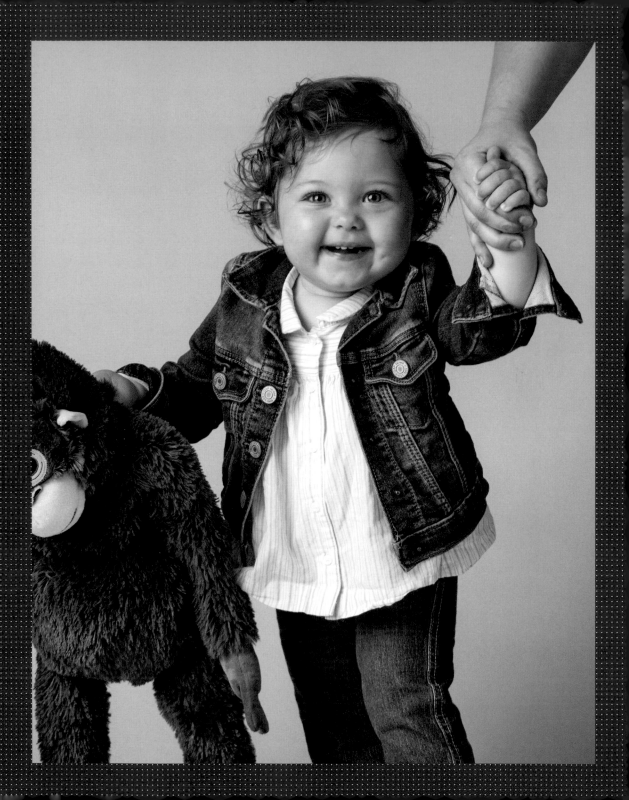

Two

A Curl Is Born

Babies & Toddlers

~~~~~~~~~~~~~~~~~~~~~~

A curly baby is born every second.

Develop your hair awareness right from the start.

Imagine this: Your sweet bundle of joy has spent nine months floating in a warm, cozy world of amniotic fluid. This soothing water bed contains nutrients, hormones, and antibodies that were custom-made just for your baby. Then it's show time: Your baby is born. Often, your baby comes out of this safe, quiet place and is placed on your chest to facilitate bonding and warm him or her up. Other times he or she is cleansed before being given to you. Either way, your baby is typically washed in a bath of man-made chemicals—often with the same ingredients that clean your greasy dishes! It's harsh but true. Shampoos and soaps contain sulfates, which are cleansing agents also found in dishwashing and laundry detergents. These chemicals are in the products used to wash your newborn's skin. The outermost layer of skin, called the epidermis, is made of natural oils, fatty lipids, and cells. They create a barrier that protects from bacteria, viruses, and other germs, acting as a shield for the healthy new skin cells underneath and warding off many common skin conditions like eczema and psoriasis. So just like

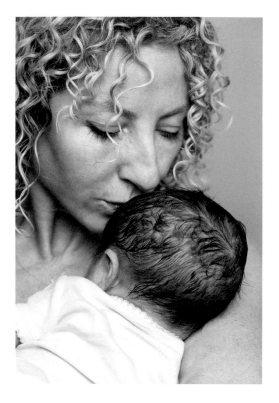

those sulfates strip grease and food particles from your plates, they strip away the skin's vital, natural oils, lipids, and antibodies, damaging the healthy skin barrier and leaving it vulnerable, exposed, dry, scaly, and itchy.

Sodium lauryl sulfate and sodium laureth sulfate, the two most commonly used chemicals in shampoos and body washes, are universally known as skin irritants that trigger allergies and are often contaminated with 1,4 dioxane, a by-product of a petrochemical process called ethoxylation. And that's not all. They are also considered probable human carcinogens. (You can find many other variations of these chemicals listed on many products' ingredient lists.) One reason they're used is to create the luxurious, frothy lather that we've all come to (wrongly) associate with being clean. The truth is this: You don't need a constant stream of suds and lather to remove minute particles known as dirt. A combination of friction, agitation, a gentle pH-balanced substance, and rinsing with water cleans most things. My point is that sulfates are not worthy of any human's skin, and especially not that belonging to a delicate newborn.

When my daughter-in-law, Veronica, went to the hospital to give birth, she actually brought a sulfate-free cleanser with her so the nurses could use it on my granddaughter, Venaih, right after she was born, to start her off on sulfate-free footing. But the nurses whisked Venaih off too quickly. Realizing that Veronica and my son Kaih had missed the chance to explain their wishes, I left the birthing room to give the cleanser to the nurses before they washed Venaih. Too late! Through the thick glass partition, I saw my minutes-old granddaughter already sudsed up in a cloud of lather. It was like a slow-motion movie where I was standing on one side of the glass pounding on the window saying, "Noooooooo!" Yet the sweet, smiling nurse could not understand my disdain through the soundproof glass. There was nothing I could do! Still clutching the bottle of sulfate-free cleanser, I went back to see my daughter-in law. Even though she had been in labor all night and was recuperating, she noticed the expression on my face.

> ## A CARE LABEL FOR CURLS
>
> I am made of organic matter. I will change based on how you treat me and various atmospheric conditions. This gives me character.
>
> Do not wash me with detergent shampoo.
>
> Use only sulfate- and silicone-free products.
>
> Do not use brushes or combs when I am dry.
>
> Do not cut me when I am wet.
>
> Do not carve, slice, thin, or razor me.
>
> Do not blow-fry me.
>
> Do not hide me under wigs and extensions.
>
> Take care of me properly and I will reward you with a gorgeous head of hair.

"What's wrong?" Veronica asked.

"They're shampooing Venaih!" I told her. Veronica had the same reaction I did! Venaih is now ten years old, and that was the first and last time she has ever had sulfate shampoo touch her skin or hair.

Unfortunately, our first minutes in the world are not the only time we're slathered in sulfates. When you're taken home from the hospital, you're often cared for with brand-name baby products that are supposed to be trusted old standbys. They are supposed to be gentle. You think, *Mom and Grandma used these. Why shouldn't I?* Although "baby" products seem innocent enough, many contain potentially dangerous ingredients—even those that have been around for many years and claim to ward off tears. Of course, most new parents don't know these products contain harmful chemicals, especially when they're sent home from the hospital or pediatrician's office with samples of them. After all, if the hospital or your doctor gave you something for your baby, it has to be safe, right? Wrong! It's just that we've been conditioned for years and years to use these products. (And who doesn't love free samples?) This sets the stage for our sulfate-filled lives and becomes all we know, the norm, as we grow from infants to preschoolers to tweens, teens, and adults. But sulfates aren't the only problem.

Many baby products have "fragrance" in their ingredient lists. In fact, look around your house and you'll see that everything from cleaning supplies to cosmetics to food products has what sounds like one simple ingredient. "However, a loophole in cosmetic labeling laws means that companies don't have to list all the chemicals that make up their fragrance," explains Jon Whelan, who wrote and directed the documentary *Stink!*, which examines the potentially toxic ingredients in our everyday products. "That one word can stand for a hundred different chemicals, many of which are derived from petroleum and are the same ones used in household cleaning products." In other words, the smell you may think is lemon is actually a blend of various synthetic ingredients engineered to have a citrus scent, even though there is nothing from a real lemon in the mix. Manufacturers can also get away with not revealing the exact components of a "fragrance" by deeming it a "trade secret." This is a huge downside for us as consumers, since some of these ingredients have been linked to issues like infertility, asthma, cancer, obesity, and learning disabilities, among others, and may be messing with our endocrine glands (not to mention what they have done to our waters)! Even if a product says it's "unscented," it just means that chemicals have been used to neutralize the odor of other ingredients. Look for "fragrance-free" instead.

> **Be vigilant in protecting your baby's hair and skin from harsh products.**

Of course, personal hygiene is very important, and we need to stay healthy and feel fresh and clean, but think about it: How dirty do babies really get? Especially in those first few months of life. They're not crawling anywhere, playing

> ### PURE DECORATION
>
> Although you may receive cute little brushes or combs as baby gifts—silver versions were popular when I had my children—you should absolutely *not* brush or comb a baby's tender scalp. Not only is it too harsh, but it's also unnecessary!

in public spaces, exposed to crowds of people, or doing much that requires us to strip them clean like we would a dirty dish or soiled clothing. Our intentions are good—we want the absolute best for our baby—but the result can be harsh and potentially damaging. Why start their precious lives that way?

I can't stress enough how important it is to pay careful attention to our children's scalps as early as possible and take a preventive approach, especially before the nutrition of the hair follicle is affected. Some of the most common infant skin conditions are eczema, also known as atopic dermatitis, psoriasis, diaper rash, and cradle cap. Diaper rash is caused by soggy diapers, and cradle cap is caused by an overgrowth of fungus and yeast that naturally occurs on the skin but has been pH altered and thus produces excess oil. Psoriasis is the result of skin cells that turn over in a matter of days rather than weeks. Eczema is caused by a damaged skin barrier. Although these conditions have other causes, they're exacerbated when skin is stripped of its natural oils and dehydrated, and it's clear that detergents, powders, and petroleum-based diaper balms are only a small part of this out-of-control and somewhat depressing global problem. It is an inconvenient truth. I can't help but think that all these skin conditions would be less common if we stopped the vicious strip-the-skin cycle. We also need to become well-educated consumers, therefore limiting the use of harsh pH-*un*balanced products made primarily with synthetic ingredients.

The CG Method for Babies and Toddlers

The CG Method can be used for toddlers as well as for infants born with a lot of hair. You will be surprised at how simple it is and that it takes the same amount of time as—or less than—a traditional cleansing routine.

- Babies and toddlers may be happier if they are facing you while you're doing the CG Method. That way you can talk to them, sing, and look into their eyes, helping to distract them. Older children, such as four- and five-year-olds, will probably be happy to face away from you and play with small bath toys while you co-wash their hair.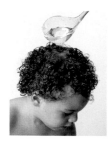

- Wet your child's hair thoroughly. If it's too difficult or unappealing to put your child's hair under running bathwater, use a plastic cup, small pail, ladle, or toy watering can.

- Apply conditioner to the pads of your fingers on one hand and rub your hands together so it gets onto the pads of the other.

- The amount of conditioner you use depends on the length and thickness of your child's hair and takes some trial and error to determine. Generally, the tighter or drier the curl, the more conditioner you need to properly hydrate and detangle. Often, the amount used will change as your child's hair becomes healthier. For example, initially you may need to use more conditioner because the hair is so dry and thirsty; with time and consistently using the CG Method, the hair will become healthier and more hydrated and will require less.

- Splay your fingers and place them directly on your child's scalp.

- Firmly but gently massage the scalp from the crown of the head to the nape of the neck. Try not to over-whirl your child's hair around his head, because too much motion can cause frizz, knots, and tangles. (I call it the "maypole effect," when hair strands, which fall off the head on a curved but fixed axis, spin when the head moves.) A bonus to this step: A light massage can be soothing to your little ones and can help them relax and unwind before bed.

- Very gently let your fingers glide downward through small sections of your child's curls. This helps you carefully untangle knots, remove loose strands that have accumulated, and organize the curls into their natural position. Don't use a comb or brush.

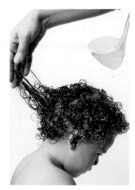

- Avoid forcefully pulling at knots and tangles. Instead, just apply more conditioner to those areas, with an added spritz of warm water to push the conditioner into the knot and detangle it more quickly.

- Rinse your child's hair with the plastic cup, pail, ladle, or small watering can or by cupping your hands together and putting them under the running water. Whether you rinse out all the conditioner or just some of it also takes trial and error as you see how the hair responds best. You can rinse out most or all of it if your child has looser curls or waves, but you typically need to leave more in the hair for coarser, tighter curls, because they tend to be drier and more frizz-prone. Children with really tight curls often don't need to rinse at all. I know that sounds unorthodox, especially since we're so conditioned (pun intended) to rinse thoroughly for fear that the hair will be weighed down or greasy. But in reality, curly hair *needs* that extra moisture to remain hydrated and frizz-free. You may also worry that leaving conditioner in will make the hair crunchy, hard, and sticky, but that should not happen when you're using products that don't contain sulfates or silicone.

- *Squeeze-quench* is a term I use to describe the process of using your hands to squeeze small sections of your child's hair in an upward motion toward the scalp. You can have your child tilt his

WHERE IT BEGAN

The word *shampoo* originated in India about three hundred years ago and described a head massage with some fragrant oil. However, the practice likely dates back centuries before that. Up until the 1940s or so, people used soap to shampoo their hair. Detergent shampooing—in which a mix of chemicals is combined with water to produce a sudsy lather—is only about eighty years old.

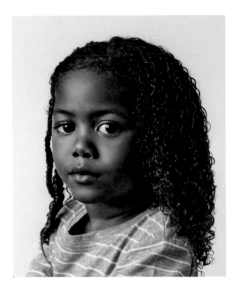

head to one side and then the other to do this or have him bend over at the waist. If you hear a luscious squishy sound, that means your mission of hydration has been accomplished. When you squeeze-quench, excess water and conditioner typically seeps through your fingers. The hair naturally drinks up and absorbs the conditioner it needs to stay properly hydrated and usually drips and releases what it doesn't. You can have a plastic container on hand to collect the milky residue. Then, if you feel like the hair needs more conditioning, you can recycle it back into your child's hair and rinse again, or you can use it after they get out of the bath or shower as a leave-in for further hydration.

- A traditional towel has fibers that can ruffle the hair's cuticle, causing frizz and disturbing each curl's natural shape.

This also applies to microfiber towels. Once your child is out of the bath or shower, use a paper towel, old T-shirt, or multipurpose towels, which you can find at Home Depot or at office supply or other big-box stores, to gently squeeze small sections of the hair upward toward the scalp. This will remove excess water and encourage each curl's natural shape.

- Try not to touch your child's curls as they dry, and tell your child not to touch them either. This may be difficult for on-the-go toddlers, so try to distract them with an art project, or by reading them a book or taking them for a drive or a walk in the stroller. Also be mindful when dressing your child, because pulling clothing on and off over the head can cause strands to disperse and frizz.

- Long or thick hair can take a while to dry, so if a bath or shower is part of your child's pre-bed routine and you don't want him going to sleep with wet hair, you can use a blow-dryer with a diffuser or a hooded helmet dryer. (These can be found online for a reasonable price.)

- For special occasions, you may want to use gel on your toddler's hair. Put a very small amount of alcohol-free, silicone-free gel in both hands, then gently rub it onto small sections of hair. Once the hair is completely dry, it may feel like it has a somewhat hard, light film of gel surrounding each curl. This is called a product cast. Once the hair is dry, you can choose to leave the hair in this cast to keep the curls a bit more protected in their shape, or you can soften and loosen the curls by opening the cast. To do this, wait until the hair is completely dry and then simply scrunch small areas of the hair upward to release the cast and curl. Then have your child tilt his head to one side, insert your fingers underneath the hair at one side of the nape of his neck, and gently shuffle your fingers at the roots to open the curls. Repeat on the other side of the head.

A FEW CURLY BABY/TODDLER NOTES

- Unless your child is extremely active or her hair is especially dirty one day, co-wash it only a few times per week, not daily. Let your child's traits and activity level determine how often. You can still bathe your child to cleanse his or her body daily; you just don't need to focus on the hair. Bonus: Think of the time you'll save!

- However, you should wash their hair after heavy sweating or swimming, because chlorine and salt water can dry the hair if not rinsed out.

- You can also spot-cleanse specific areas of the hair if necessary between cleansing days. (See the recipe for What Knots? on page 162.)

HOW TO HANDLE BEDHEAD

When your little one wakes up from a nap or you pick her up after she has been lying

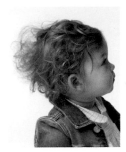

down during playtime (like on a play mat) or from sitting in a car seat or stroller, the hair in the back can appear matted and messy. The following can help it spring back into shape and, when used from your child's early days, can help prevent knots and start good hair habits for the future.

1. Fill a spray bottle with Co-Wash in a Bottle (see the recipe on page 170).

2. Shake well before using.

3. Spritz the bedhead hair with the watered-down conditioner.

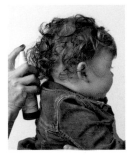

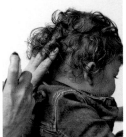

4. Gently comb it through with your fingers.

5. If needed, scrunch gently. Let dry without touching.

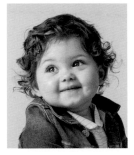

WHAT TO DO?

When a baby is born, his or her skin is covered in a naturally occurring substance rich in fat called the vernix caseosa, also known as vernix. This waxy, cheeselike coating is produced in the last trimester of pregnancy. It is believed to play a protective role during fetal development, and, as your baby transitions from the womb to the

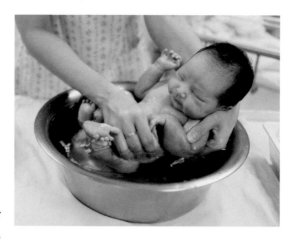

real world, it possibly helps to prevent water loss, regulate body temperature, and enhance immunity. Ideally, you should bring a sulfate- and fragrance-free cleansing product with you to the hospital when you go into labor, as well as pure sweet almond oil, and insist that the nurses and other hospital staff use it to cleanse your newborn child. (If possible, discuss this with your doctor, midwife, partner, and/or labor nurse in advance.) To gently remove the fatty layer that covers the scalp, the staff can saturate the baby's scalp with the pure sweet almond oil and leave it on while washing the baby's body with a sulfate-free cleanser. Then they can gently cleanse the scalp with this same sulfate-free product to remove the oil. It's highly unlikely that any of the fatty coating will remain after the first bath, but if it does, you may add more oil and leave it on the scalp until the next day.

Once your baby is home, you can continue to use the pure sweet almond oil (also good for diaper rash and other skin irritations) and wash your baby's scalp, hair, and body every day or every other day with products that are 100 percent free of sulfates, silicone, and fragrance. If you've been living in a shampoo-filled world, at first it may be hard *not* to see a frothy lather or a tub full of bubbles. You might not think you're getting the baby clean without them. But trust me, you are. What really removes debris particles is movement and friction. It's the gentle movement and slight agitation of your finger pads on your baby's scalp, hair, and body that lift and dislodge particles, which you can then flush away with water. Pat the skin and blot the hair dry, and apply a little pure sweet almond or olive oil to retain moisture.

Though it's typically used for toddlers on up, babies with a lot of hair may benefit from the CG Method.

Remember this: Our children and their curls depend on us. We need to lead the way!

HAPPY HAIR FROM AGES TWO TO FIVE YEARS OLD

Whereas babies' lack of mobility means they tend to stay pretty clean, toddlers are the total opposite. Excited by their new independence, they can't wait to get into things no matter how hard we try to watch over them. As a result, they are naturally skilled at getting filthy in mere minutes, taste-testing everything—especially what's not supposed to go in their mouths, such as small toys, grit, and sand—and

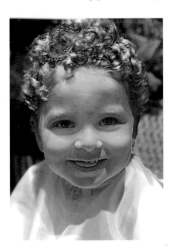

touching anything and everything. And often they can do this all while having a tantrum! That said, this amazing, unbounded curiosity about the world around them makes the toddler years the perfect time to plant the seeds for a future of healthy curl care. Talking your child through their hair-cleansing steps and being as diligent and consistent as possible early on, nurture positive hair habits for life as well as good overall hygiene. This not only benefits their hair, and you, but also prepares them for years later when it's time to bathe and shower themselves.

TALK CURLY TO ME

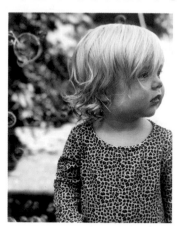

Experts suggest that the more you talk to your baby and toddler, the richer her vocabulary will be. Bath time is the perfect time to talk through the hair-cleansing routine, to engage your child, distract her, expand her vocabulary, and teach her about hair care. Older toddlers love to ask questions, so you'll often hear, "But why? Why?" For example, just a year earlier, your child may not have noticed you were washing her hair, but now she may ask what you're putting in it or where the water goes. Engage this curiosity by explaining things you do, including how and why you're so carefully caring for her curls. This is a great way to make this kind of curl care a habit.

LET THEM HELP

"I do it. I do it" is a phrase you'll start to hear as your toddler gets older. She wants to do things herself, partly because of a new sense of independence and partly because her fine-motor skills are developing. She wants to walk without holding your hand and to pour her own glass of juice. She may also want to cleanse her own body and hair in the tub. Although she may not do it the way *you* would or according to the CG Method, let her think she's doing it herself by giving her small tasks such as pouring the conditioner into your hands or cupping her hands to rinse. Praising your child's efforts helps boost her confidence and inspires her to be even more independent. And, of course, you're planting the seeds for a healthy CG life!

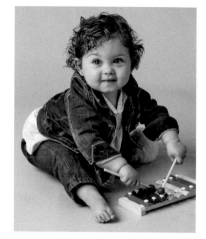

Curly Kid Inspiration

Liliana Caracóis Saudáveis

At just four years old, my daughter, Lia, already knows how to take care of her curls by herself and explains the CG Method to others. Putting her hair in the pineapple is part of her bedtime routine, right after brushing her teeth. And she loves sleeping with a satin pillowcase. Just one year ago, before we started the CG Method, her hair got tangled very easily and we had to wash it almost every day just to detangle it. Now she washes it two to three times a week.

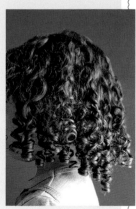

CO-WASHING AND DETANGLING KNOTS

Because your kids are in constant motion, knots—especially at the nape of the neck—can be a part of daily life. (That said, I have clients who have been using the CG Method since the day their babies were born and have never seen a knot.) This technique is the ideal way to detangle without damage. It's also great for spot cleansing the hair between washes. The analogy I often use for this approach is to look at the hair like you would a favorite dry clean-only dress or coat. You don't wash it each time you wear it, right? If you did, it would get worn-out very quickly. Overwashing wears out hair and makes it drier and more tangled. Nevertheless, you should spot clean fabric if you spill something on it. You can do the same thing with hair, especially small tangles that you want to eliminate before they turn into major let's-cut-them-out knots.

• Examine the entire landscape of your child's hair for any knots and tangles. These are often hidden under the canopy of the hair near the nape of the neck or in the middle of the back of the head.

Advice from a Stylist

Melissa Stites, There Once Was a Curl Salon in Southgate, MI

Having red curly hair was a double whammy when I was growing up. It was the beginning of every compliment and every insult—adults loved it; kids hated it.

When I was six, in an effort to control my hair, my mom took me to a swanky salon. I sat there crying with my head hanging down, watching and feeling my long hair fall to the floor. When it was over, the hair that had been down to my lower back was boy-short.

At sixteen years old, I decided to take control of the situation. So I went to beauty school and graduated before the year was up. I cut all my hair off into a pixie cut so people would see me and the work I did, *not* just my big red hair. People loved what I did, and I loved doing it. I got invited to slumber parties to do the girls' hair. I was asked to come to parties early so I could do people's hair. I did hair for all of my friends' weddings. When other kids were getting in trouble for smoking, I was getting in trouble for using perm solution.

In 2000, a curly-haired friend made a video of herself getting a haircut in New York from a curly hair specialist. As the stylist cut her hair, I saw what he was doing, and the way he was explaining it made sense to me. I started doing the same thing for myself and my curly clients. The transformations were life-changing.

I now have more than two thousand clients and am head over heels in love with my curls and everyone else's. Introducing women and children to their natural beauty inside and out has become my life's passion.

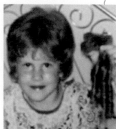

- Isolate one knot. It may sound tedious, but you need to work on each one individually so that you untangle it without tearing the hair or causing breakage.

- On dry hair, use your fingers to saturate the knot with a silicone- and sulfate-free conditioner, or put the conditioner and warm water in a spray bottle and spritz the area until it's wet.

- Let the conditioner soak into the hair, using your fingers to squeeze it in further. This will protect the hair from tearing when you start to untangle and will help the strands separate more easily.

- Once the hair feels sufficiently hydrated and softened, isolate the knot between both thumbs and forefingers and gently loosen and release each strand of tangled hair.

- Be gentle. This is the equivalent of getting a knot out of a chain necklace or detaching a bracelet that's stuck on a favorite piece of clothing. You would never tug and tear those delicate items, so don't do it to the hair, or it will tear and fray.

- There is no need to rinse out the conditioning milk when you are finished. It may look odd at first, because you've got two competing textures of the hair—one wet and one dry—lying on top of each other. But see it through. The hair will dry more quickly because only small parts of it are saturated. This bit of conditioner will also refresh the surrounding curls.

- Many mommy blogs suggest traditional shampooing and then conditioning before trying to detangle a knot. But sulfate-filled shampoo actually makes the knots and tangles worse. Also, never use a brush or comb to unsnarl the hair, because that just fuses the open cuticles of each strand so they attach to one another like Velcro.

- Untangling a knot as soon as you see it will save you time and energy in the long run. Having to deal with cumulative knots is harder and can result in major breakage and damage. It can also be overwhelming when you feel the only option is cutting them out—an outcome no one will be happy with.

HAIR AND SELF-ESTEEM

As we know by now, children—including young toddlers—take in just about everything we say and do and are quick to pick up on prejudices of all kinds. This includes comments about them and their physical appearance, even a casual remark. Many curly girls and boys I've met recount painful words that an adult used to describe their hair. And if it wasn't words

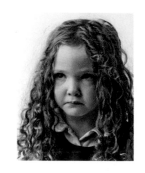

that hurt these children, it was an adult's actions and frustrations that sent the message loud and clear that curly/wavy/coily hair was something to control and hide, not embrace and love. Their hair was not okay. In turn, many of these curlies interpreted this to mean that *they* were not okay.

People I meet who are well into their forties, fifties, or sixties still share their hair-shaming stories from when they were children and teens as though those experiences happened just yesterday. It makes me sad that they still carry the burden of these memories. It's clear that words affect us more than we realize at the time they're spoken. I think this could be why straightening, blowouts, and weaves have become so prevalent.

EVOLUTIONARY LEAPS

The skin is the body's largest organ, one that has been through many adaptations since we started walking upright. Hair, an evolutionary development from reptile scales, is adapted from the same materials found in claws, horns, and nails, yet it has the same molecular structure as fur, wool, and feathers. Its main purpose is to preserve heat in the body and protect it. Of course, it also promotes individuality.

Of course, many parents and guardians aren't always aware that they are projecting their frustrations onto their little ones. I would like to think that their motivation is to benefit their children by helping them feel good about themselves and look well kept. I don't blame those parents. We are only human, just trying to get through our busy days, and don't even realize that what we are saying may be hurtful and everlasting. But our kids listen and internalize these negative comments, which can really affect their self-esteem. My point is that we have a big responsibility to choose our words and actions carefully, both avoiding negative comments and making self-esteem-boosting remarks whenever the opportunity arises. This helps cultivate a positive self-image. I suggest talking to your children about their natural curls as if they have a beautiful garden living on top of their heads. I always like to use

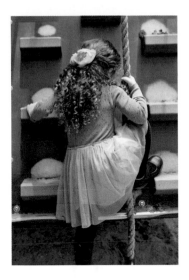

nature analogies, but if comparing hair to a garden isn't right for you and your child, just choose another positive analogy. It also helps to point out other kids and

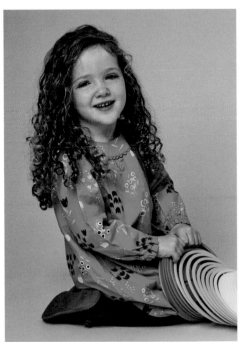

adults who have beautiful curls so your child sees natural hair in the world around her, and to talk about how much you love your own curls if you have them. If you have naturally straight hair, find your child a curly-haired role model to connect with. Many of us curly girls and guys might have avoided years of agony, especially during our adolescence, if we'd only had a curly mentor. These conversations with your child will change as he or she gets older, but starting them early plants seeds about the importance of the care and appreciation of your natural hair.

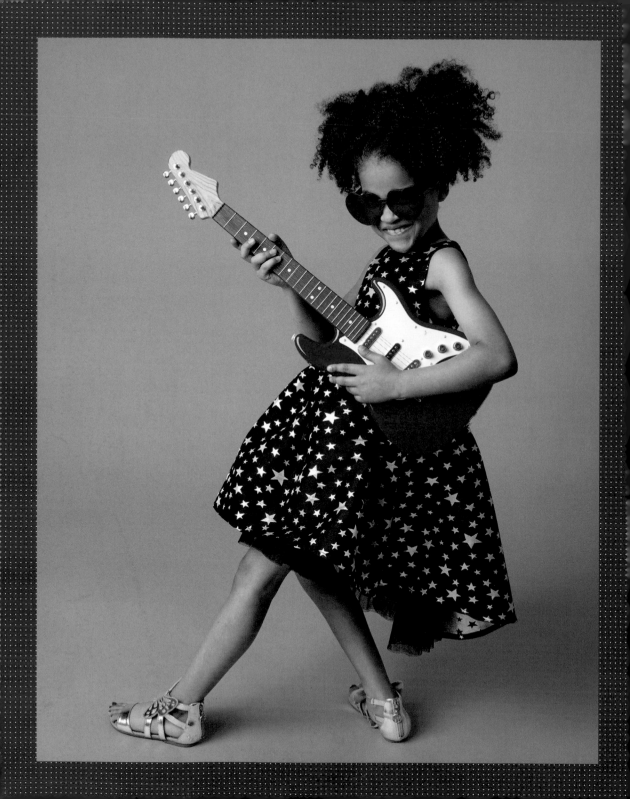

Three

Grade School Curls

Ages 5–10

Your curls are nothing without you.
Care for them and you will love them for life!

ntering grade school is an exciting time for your child. It brings new friends, adventures, and independence. It also brings lice, tangles, and foreign matter like gum and paint that get stuck in your child's strands. The solutions for all of these issues typically involve touching and fussing with the hair, combs, and special products—things that are no-no's for curls. This chapter will help you remedy those problems *and* keep curls healthy and looking their best. We'll also discuss cleansing your grade-schooler's hair and transitioning from washing your child's hair to him doing it all by himself. These grade school years are also the time when children may start to notice that their curly, wavy, kinky hair is not the same as their friends'. Teaching them how to co-wash, care for, and love their curls, waves, and coils will help them care for and love themselves too!

The CG Method for Grade School Kids

These directions are aimed at the parent, but your child may be ready to do this method solo, as pictured here. Support this! Just check in to be sure the steps are being followed correctly.

Wet your child's hair thoroughly. If your child is taking showers rather than baths, just have her stand under the 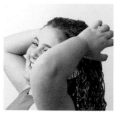 running water until her hair is wet. In the bath, use a plastic cup, small pail, or ladle or have her put her head under the running water.

Apply conditioner to the pads of your fingers on one hand and rub your hands together.

The amount of conditioner you use depends on the length and thickness of your child's 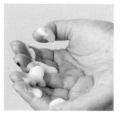 hair. Generally, the tighter or drier the curl, the more you need to properly hydrate and detangle. Often, the amount used will change as your child's hair becomes healthier.

Initially you may need to use more conditioner because the hair is so dry and thirsty; with time and consistency, it will become healthier and more hydrated and will require less.

Splay your fingers and place them directly on your child's scalp. Firmly but gently massage the scalp from the 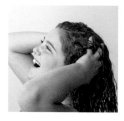 crown of the head to the nape of the neck. Try not to whirl the hair around because too much motion can cause frizz, knots, and tangles.

Gently let your fingers glide downward through your child's curls. This helps you carefully untangle 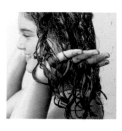 knots, remove loose strands that have accumulated, and organize the curls into their natural position. Don't use a comb or brush.

If your child has long hair, scrunch small sections of curls up toward the scalp.

Gliding your fingers through longer hair in the previous step can make curls stretch out, so scrunching afterward encourages their natural shape.

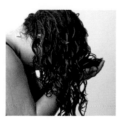

- Avoid forcefully pulling at knots and tangles. Instead, just apply more conditioner to those areas, with an added spritz of warm water to push the conditioner into the knot and detangle it more quickly. If your child is doing his or her own hair, tell them not to tug too hard at a serious knot and instead ask someone else to help them. Explain to them that it's hard to detangle a knot you can't see, and you risk tearing the hair.

- If your child is in the shower, have her step away from standing directly under the running water and tell her to rinse her hair by cupping her hands together, putting them under the running water, and then pouring the water onto her head. I call this method "the baptism." Standing directly under the running water can rinse away too much conditioner and can also disturb the curls' natural shape. If your child is in the bath, you can use cupped hands or a plastic cup, pail, or ladle. Deciding whether to rinse out all the conditioner or just some of it also takes some trial and error as you see how the hair responds best. You can rinse out most or all of it if your child has looser curls or waves.

For coarser, tighter curls, leave in more conditioner, because those curls tend to be drier and more frizz-prone. Some people with really tight curls don't need to rinse at all. I know that sounds unorthodox, especially since we're so conditioned (pun intended) to rinse thoroughly for fear that the hair will be weighed down or greasy. But in reality, curly hair *needs* that extra moisture to remain hydrated and frizz-free. You may also worry that leaving conditioner in will make the hair crunchy, hard, and sticky, but that should not happen when you're using products that don't contain sulfates and silicone.

- *Squeeze-quench* is a term I use to describe the process of using your hands to squeeze small sections of your child's hair in an upward motion toward the scalp. You can have your child tilt his head to one side and then the other or have him bend over at the waist. If you hear a luscious squishy sound, that means your mission of hydration has been accomplished. When you squeeze-quench, a milky residue of excess water and conditioner typically seeps through your fingers. The hair naturally drinks up and absorbs the conditioner it needs to stay properly hydrated and usually drips and releases what it doesn't. Have a plastic container on hand to collect the milky residue. If you feel like the hair needs more conditioning, you can pour it back into your child's hair and rinse again or leave it in the hair.

A traditional terry-cloth towel has fibers that can ruffle the hair's cuticle, causing frizz and disturbing each 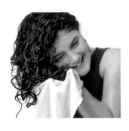 curl's natural shape. With a traditional towel, you also can't feel the water content in the hair and how much water you want to remove or keep in. This also applies to microfiber towels. So once your child is out of the bath or shower, use a paper towel, an old T-shirt, or multipurpose towels, which you can find at Home Depot or at office supply or other big-box stores, to gently squeeze small sections of the hair upward toward the scalp. This will remove excess water and encourage each curl's natural shape.

Try not to touch your child's curls as they dry and tell your child not to touch them either. Also, 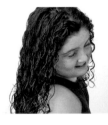 have her dress carefully, because pulling clothing on and off over her head can cause strands to disperse and frizz. If you need to distract your child from touching her hair, play a game, do an art project, or bake together. This keeps little hands too busy to fuss with curls.

Long or thick hair can take a while to dry, so if a bath or shower is part of your child's pre-bed routine and you don't want her going to sleep with wet hair, you can use a blow-dryer with a diffuser or hooded helmet dryer (reasonably priced online).

If you use styling gel on your child's hair (at this age, it's probably just for special occasions), the hair may feel like it is in a product cast—a light film of gel surrounding each curl—once it's completely dry. Some people like to leave the hair in this cast and let it open up naturally. This is great for preserving the hair for special occasions later in the day or if it's raining.

Other times, you may want your child's curls to look more open. In that case, once the hair is completely dry, simply scrunch small areas of the hair upward to release the cast and curl. Then insert your fingers underneath the hair at one side of the nape of your child's neck. Have her tilt her head to that side while you gently shuffle your fingers at the roots to open the curls. Repeat on the other side of the head.

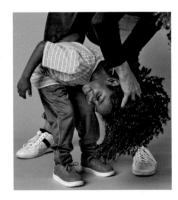

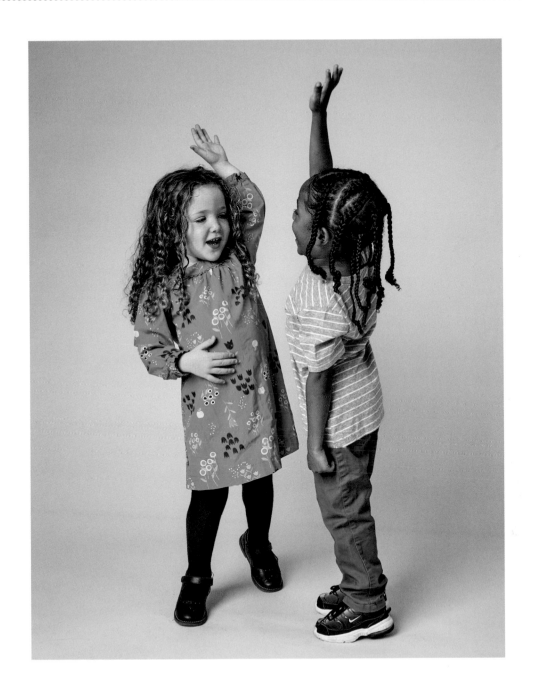

PRECLEANSE CONDITIONING

This precleanse conditioning is great for long, thick, dry hair and hair that doesn't get wet easily. It's also good if you live in an area with hard water. It creates a barrier so the hair does not absorb the minerals in hard water that can make your hair feel rough and tangled.

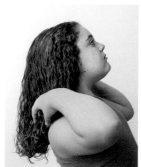

• Apply a silicone-free conditioner to dry hair to moisten it.

• Allow it to absorb for at least ten minutes. If you're worried about the conditioner dripping while you wait, have your child put on a shower cap or drape a towel around her shoulders. However, when conditioner alone is applied to dry hair, you usually won't get many drips because the thirsty hair will soak it up.

• After at least ten minutes, have your child get into the tub or shower and wet her hair. When she rinses out this preconditioning treatment, you will notice how quickly the water penetrates, immediately wetting and softening the hair. This is especially effective for hair that repels water and never feels wet enough before applying cleansers or conditioners. After using this preconditioning method for a while, you will begin to feel true hydration taking place in the hair and it will become easier to care for.

• After this, go on to the usual CG Method that's detailed earlier: Apply conditioner, gently pull it through the hair, rinse, squeeze-quench, blot dry, and then air-dry if possible.

PASSING THE CLEANSING TORCH

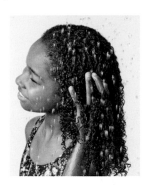

All kids are different. Some want to do their hair themselves as early as age six or seven; others want an adult to do it until they're teens. When your child does it herself, it may not be perfect, but give her a lot of leeway and encouragement. The last thing you want to do is add stress to the process or discourage her. Remember, this is a great step toward independence! That said, once your child is left to her own devices (and alone in the bathroom), bad hair habits can start and then may last a lifetime. Initially, you may have to step in and do some coaching. This happened with my son Dylan. Soon after he started cleansing his curls on his own, his thick red curly hair looked oily. Then I saw clumps of conditioner in it after he got out of the shower. I also noticed an odor. This can be caused by product buildup and not massaging the scalp enough or at all and thus not helping to lift away dirt and oils. Dylan was not taking care of his hair correctly, so it was time for a one-on-one lesson on proper cleansing and rinsing! I had Dylan put on his bathing suit and get in the shower. Then I coached him. "That's not enough conditioner! Use more! Move it around! Okay, rinse! You missed a spot! Now scrunch!" It may not sound like much fun, but the difference it made in his hair was remarkable. And the difference it made in his confidence is

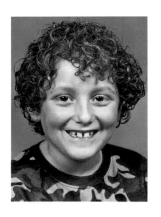

hard to put into words. He finally owned—and loved—his head full of bright, hydrated, and defined curls. Simply have your child get into the shower or bath and guide them using the steps in the CG Method. You may need to help out at first or check in every once in a while, but luckily the steps are straightforward enough that they will catch on, and typically at this stage, kids are motivated to be independent. Over time, you can keep improving your child's technique.

You probably will need to guide your children in how often they should wash their hair, depending on their activities. Each child is different. Changes in weather also have a big effect. To determine if your child is cleansing too much or too little, look at his hair and scalp after he gets out of the shower.

• If your child's hair and/or scalp appears oily, the natural instinct is to wash the hair more often. Instead, reduce the number of times per week you co-wash by one (for example, if the hair is normally co-washed four times a week, do it three times). See how the hair reacts. If there's no change, cut out another co-wash and see if that helps reduce the amount of oil.

• If your child's hair is dull, dry, and/or shedding an unusual amount, add one or two co-washes per week until it looks shinier and more hydrated.

• Another issue could be using too much styling product or the wrong conditioner and leaving it in. That won't happen with sulfate-, silicone-, and alcohol-free styling products.

GUM AND OTHER FOREIGN OBJECTS

Glue, paint, and gum that get caught in the hair take a little extra effort to remove.

• For gum, rub the area with an ice cube until the sticky mess hardens. That may begin to dislodge it. An ice cube works best with a small amount of gum and when not too much hair is tangled.

• If glue or paint is the issue, try dipping the affected hair into a cup of apple cider vinegar or witch hazel, which acts like a solvent to break down the bond between the hair and the glue or paint. Let it soak as you gently rub it with your fingers to loosen it. It leaves a strong odor behind, but that will be remedied after cleansing and/or conditioning.

Advice from a Stylist

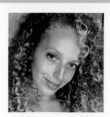

Joleigh Wynter, owner of Curl Talk Salon in London

My mum didn't have curls, so my hair was a struggle for her. Once-a-week wash day was so traumatic that I would actually hide the brush. Now that I have three curly-haired daughters, I maintain their hair on a daily basis, so washing it is quick, fun, and painless.

I never really felt welcome in salons when I was growing up and couldn't ignore the look of dread from the stylists when I walked in with my big curls. All my haircuts ended in tears. I became obsessed with understanding curls and determined to master them myself. I searched the internet for answers and was given *Curly Girl: The Handbook*. It was a major light-bulb moment for me. After that, I started cutting my own hair dry. Then I began to cut my friends' hair, and word spread. Soon I was trimming friends of friends' hair and their mums' and *their* friends' hair. The fact that people would trust a self-trained teenager over a professional stylist shows how much salons did not understand curls. The smiles and happiness I would bring to people sparked my passion for becoming a curl specialist.

Years later I opened Curl Talk Salon, the first curly-hair-only salon in the heart of Bricklane, London. Kids as young as three years old come in saying they don't like their curls. We give them the right haircut and show them exactly how to care for their hair so every child leaves with a smile and the confidence that they can style their own hair. My mission is to empower curlies to embrace themselves, change their hairdressing experience, and live up to their curls' true potential.

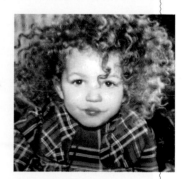

- Another option is to apply about half a teaspoon each of conditioner and vinegar (depending on the size of the substance stuck in the hair). If you're not able to work the tangle out with your fingers, try to gently break up the gum, paint, or glue mass with the end of a knitting needle.

- Some people use peanut butter to dislodge gum, but I have not tried it. I believe it works on the theory that the oil will loosen the gum's stickiness. But it may not be the ideal option during school or camp or other times your child will be around other kids, because one in fifty children has a peanut allergy.

MODEL BEHAVIOR

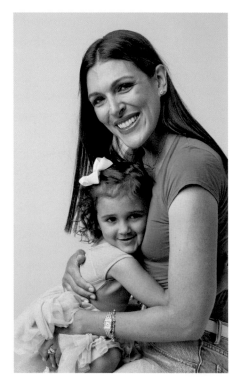

If you're a mom who blows out and flat-irons her hair, you are, unfortunately, showing your child that Mom doesn't accept her curls. Without saying a word, you're telling her that *her* natural hair isn't good enough either. *If curly is beautiful, wouldn't Mom like her curls too?* your child may think. This brings me to another point: If you are still in denial of your natural hair texture and you have a curly kid, it's time to start loving what you were born with. Whether you like it or not, you are your child's first beauty consultant. If you live with and love your curls, so will your child. But if you hide them—even if you never actually talk about straightening your hair or not liking your curls—you'll send a message that curls are something to cover up

After this photo shoot, Ruby's mom, Rebeca, was inspired to stop straightening her hair and begin her journey back to her own natural curls.

and be ashamed of. Many of my curly clients recall mothers who sent that message, making them believe that straight hair was beautiful and curly hair was ugly. That is what happened with Tia Williams, who was happy with the thrice-yearly relaxers and the weekly blowouts she had been doing for as long as she could remember. As Tia puts it, she comes from the "relaxer at puberty era." Her straight hair was also easy, and she never worried about it unless she was somewhere near the equator. That is, until she gave birth to Lina—a black, Dominican, Panamanian girl with curls. Lina was only three years old when she started saying that she wanted "princess" hair (i.e., straight like Rapunzel's) and that she hated her curls. She and Tia had a conversation that went something like this:

Lina: You have long hair like Rapunzel. I don't have any hair.

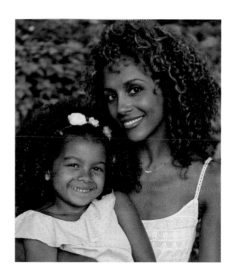

Tia: You have stunningly beautiful curls. And guess what? Mommy has curls too. I just, um, straighten them . . . which is silly, because curls are so beautiful.

Lina (*looking skeptical*): You don't have curls. Me and Daddy have curls, and he's a boy. I don't like curls.

Tia said that's when her heart broke. *She already doesn't like her curls? At three years old?* she thought. It didn't matter that two of Lina's best friends and her auntie Lauren had curls or that Tia bought her curly-haired dolls and books with curly-haired heroines.

Curly Kid Inspiration

Mindi Morris

I've always struggled with my wavy/curly hair. In elementary school, I opted for the modified mullet; in middle school, I used a lot of Dippity-Do and hair spray. The result was crunchy hair and ceiling-high bangs! In high school, I tried to straighten my hair with a clothes iron. I singed it so badly that I had to walk through the halls at school reeking of sulfur!

Now I've got two curly-haired kids. My fourteen-year-old son, Drew, has always embraced his corkscrews and likes the way they make him stand out in a crowd. Although he's typically an introvert, his face lights up when someone compliments them (though he isn't so happy when someone can't resist touching them). On the other hand, my eleven-year-old daughter, Grace, is engaged in a war against her curls, fighting them at every turn. Although I hate to make it a gender issue, I do think tween/teen females think they need to have a certain look to fit in and are more influenced by what is portrayed as beautiful on TV and in social media and print.

I remember feeling the same way as a teen and even into adulthood. I've had to work hard to find a mantra for myself. When I feel like I'm failing, I repeat, "I am enough." When I compare myself to everyone who is doing anything better than me, "I am enough." Because of this, I can finally, in my forties, leave the house without makeup just as easily as I can walk out with a made-up face. It's why I can wash my hair, throw some gel in it, and waltz out to let it air-dry instead of trying to force it into something it's never going to be. It's why now I can be me. Because I am enough. And I am trying with every ounce of my being to teach my kids that lesson earlier than I learned it myself.

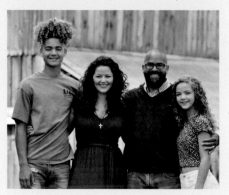

"None of it mattered," Tia recalls. "Every little girl wants to look like her *mommy*." The final straight-haired straw came one night when Lina wasn't feeling well and got into bed with Tia.

"She spread my hair on her shoulder and stroked it until she fell asleep—but not before murmuring, 'So soft; my hair's not soft,'" Tia explains. "I was devastated." Devastated, but she snapped back to reality. At that moment, Tia knew she had to embrace her natural hair texture. "There was no way I could teach her to love her gorgeous spirals while I was chemically straightening mine. The nerve of me, trying to convince her that her texture is pretty when I beat my own into submission! It's my job to do everything I can to help my daughter feel strong, whole, and confident, and as black and brown women know, hair hate is a soul killer. I wanted to show Lina that curls are awesome and a part of our fierceness! Mothers are our first beauty icons. My thinking was, if she believes *my* hair is pretty, she'll think hers is too—and it worked." Although it took two years for Tia's hair to return to its natural curly state, she's never regretted her decision, and it truly changed Lina's perception of her own hair.

"Curly hair can be complicated sometimes, but it's also cool—with a lot of personality and character—as long as you know what to do with it," says Lina at age eleven. "It's special and I'm glad I have it."

LICE BE GONE

Few things send a parent or guardian into a panic more than the school nurse calling to tell them their child has head lice. I'll be honest: Lice are not fun, not pretty, not easy. But getting lice *is* par for the course during grade school. If your child gets through these years without it, congrats. But unfortunately, nobody is immune to lice. An estimated 6 million to 12 million infestations occur each year in American children ages three to eleven, according to the Centers for Disease

Control. Lice are also common among the caregivers of preschool and elementary school children and those who live with them. This makes sense since lice are passed from one person to another through head-to-head contact or sharing things like pillows, hairbrushes, hats, barrettes, clothing, scarves, and so on. (And it's a myth that you can't get lice if you have color-treated hair, so everyone's strands are fair game.) Some research reveals that girls get this itchy head condition more often than boys. But when it's *your* child who's got lice, studies and statistics don't matter.

The good news is that you *can* treat lice and nits (the eggs) at home—no expensive professional services needed—and there are several things you can do to prevent them. Again, lice are no fun for anyone, but curlies especially can suffer from the harsh ingredients typically found in lice products, the silicone in inexpensive drugstore conditioners usually recommended for lice removal, and all the combing and handling. Lice removal is the *only* time I will ever recommend you use a comb of any sort on a wavy, curly, or coily child or adult.

Two things to ease your mind: The main issue with lice is itchiness, not the spread of any diseases, and getting lice has *nothing* to do with hygiene. I think it's important that your kids realize that there's nothing wrong with them just because they have lice. In today's world we have a heightened sensitivity to kids' feelings, but I've had clients tell me horror stories about lice checks in front of the whole class and mortifying moments when they were told they had lice. Apparently, these little buggers have been around for centuries. Lice were found on the hair of a mummified queen who

LICE NO-NO'S

Some lice-removal techniques found online or elsewhere suggest using silicone- and sulfate-filled shampoos and conditioners, petroleum jelly, coconut oil, or mayonnaise. I *do not* recommend any of these things. Sulfate- and silicone-filled cleansers and conditioners can dry out and tangle hair while creating a watertight coating that makes the lice harder to remove.

had been encased in wax. Lice survive off the blood from our heads and can hide well, especially in curly hair that has a lot of texture to nestle into. By the time you notice your child scratching her head (or find yourself scratching too), those little bugs have really made themselves at home in the landscape of your child's hair. The only solution is to eradicate the lice and their eggs one nit at a time. And I mean that. You have to pull them out individually, but I'll show you how to do it as painlessly as possible.

> ### HAIR, THERE, AND EVERYWHERE
>
> Make sure to check everyone in the family, kids *and* adults. Lice may be small, but they spread easily, especially on surfaces like fabric couches, bedding, and clothes. Launder sheets, pillowcases, blankets, clothing, stuffed animals, and anything else that may have come in contact with the heads of those affected in hot water above 130°F, which will kill the lice and nits.

If your child has really long or thick hair, your first thought after the nurse calls may be to shave it all off. But that's not necessary (and would be even more upsetting to many kids). First, take a deep breath. Cry if you must. It *is* work, but the only way around this dilemma is through it (the hair) so the lice don't spread to you and others who come in contact with your child. Tell anyone who has been around your child in the past few days that they need to check their hair. Do not take your child for a haircut, since it's considered a health code violation. And then get to work.

Today, plenty of lice-treatment products are available. Some use natural ingredients like tea tree oil and are labeled "nontoxic" and "pesticide-free," but some well-known, over-the-counter lice shampoos contain pyrethrins (pesticides derived from chrysanthemum flowers), permethrin (an insecticide), and piperonyl butoxide (a man-made ingredient in pesticides). Yes, pesticides! There are also stronger prescription products, such as ivermectin and spinosad (Natroba). In my opinion, you don't need to use harsh chemicals, especially when they will be on the hair for a long time, sitting very close to your child's eyes, nose, and mouth. These ingredients can also dry out already-thirsty curls, upping your chances of frizz and distorted curl shapes. I have several curly clients who, after getting lice from their young children, used traditional lice-treatment shampoos and told me their hair was not the same, both in thickness and texture, for a long time afterward.

In my experience, the most important ingredients in getting rid of lice are your effort and a lice comb, available at most drugstores or online. This all-important comb has very fine teeth so it can effectively remove lice and nits, which are very small and hard to see. Harsher chemical treatments claim to suffocate the lice, but apparently, they just stun them and make them slower and easier to catch on the comb. The pure essential oil and conditioner treatment described below can do those things too. Obviously, the choice of treatment is your own, but if you opt for the one here, which works for all hair types from thick to fine, long to short, do it every day for a week. For two weeks after that, check the hair daily to make sure the lice are gone. If you see any lice or nits, take a deep breath and repeat the treatment every day for another week. And let me just say this: If you need this treatment, my sympathy goes out to you. But know everything will be all right and you will get through this. Get all the items on this list, get into a consistent rhythm, and just get started.

YOU'LL NEED THE FOLLOWING ITEMS

• Two or three fine-tooth lice combs. You need a few so you can rotate and sterilize one while using the other.

• A kettle of simmering hot water for sterilization.

• Essential oil. My favorite is tea tree oil.

- A sulfate- and silicone-free conditioner. Although I *never* suggest you use any products that contain silicone, it is very important to use a silicone-free conditioner, because this ingredient can create a film on the hair that can repel water, making the lice harder to remove.

- Disposable gloves.

- A stainless-steel spray bottle containing hot water. The heat of the water in the spray helps soften the hair, making it easier to catch, stun, or kill the nits.

- Household bleach, Dettol, or rubbing alcohol.

- Three containers: one for the lice application mix, one filled with hot water and household bleach or other antiseptic in which to deposit and rinse the combed-out lice, and one with plain hot water to remove the bleach-antiseptic solution on the comb before using it again on the next section of hair.

- A black plastic disposable tablecloth to wrap around your child's upper body so you can see any remaining nits. A large disposable garbage bag with a hole in the bottom to go over the head also works well.

HOW TO

- Wet hair thoroughly and wash it with a sulfate-free cleanser or conditioner. Then rinse it out completely.

- Sit your little one in front of her favorite movie or video game to help create a distraction, because this process can take a long time. Even better, use this time to catch up. (Okay, your kids won't go for it. But maybe it will work for a little while; then you can opt for screen time.)

- Have the bowl with piping-hot water and bleach or an antiseptic solution ready nearby to rinse off the comb.

- Add ten to fifteen drops of the essential oil of your choice to a cup of silicone-free conditioner and mix well. You may need more than a cup for longer hair. The conditioner will soften and protect the hair from damage and prepare it for the methodical and focused lice-be-gone comb-out.

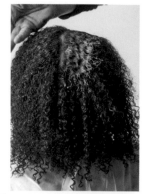

- Apply the conditioner mix to hair. The idea here is to cover every strand with the conditioning treatment so that the lice are forced to slow down or become immobilized.

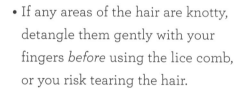
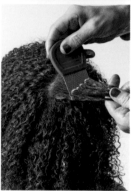

- If any areas of the hair are knotty, detangle them gently with your fingers *before* using the lice comb, or you risk tearing the hair.

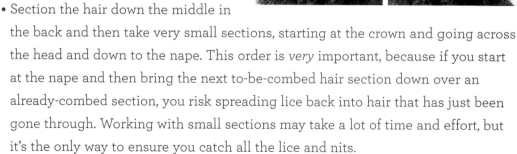

- Section the hair down the middle in the back and then take very small sections, starting at the crown and going across the head and down to the nape. This order is *very* important, because if you start at the nape and then bring the next to-be-combed hair section down over an already-combed section, you risk spreading lice back into hair that has just been gone through. Working with small sections may take a lot of time and effort, but it's the only way to ensure you catch all the lice and nits.

- Comb each section downward starting at the scalp, gathering the lice and nits in the conditioner mix along the way.

- When you get to the end of the hair in one section, use a gloved hand or plastic bag to thoroughly rinse, scrape, and wipe off the comb into the bowl with hot water and bleach-antiseptic solution.

- Then place the comb into the bowl of piping-hot water to sterilize it while you use a different lice comb on the next section. This keeps you from putting the lice and nits you've extracted back into the hair.

- You will need gloves or something to protect your hands when you retrieve the comb from the bowl for the next section.

- Periodically, spritz the hair with the spray bottle containing warm water; this helps keep the conditioner fluid and wet, making it easier for the comb to glide through the hair.

WARD OFF LICE

To prevent lice from infesting your life in the future, try these tips:

- Teach your children that they should never share combs, pillows, helmets, and hats with other kids, since these items, among others, can pass lice from one child to another.

- Make sure to regularly wash that one cuddly toy they take with them wherever they go.

- Believe it or not, my three kids never had lice during their school years. I credit my homemade lavender cleansing spray, which I'd religiously spritz on them before school each morning to refresh their tresses or unravel a knot or two. It is also known to repel lice. (See the Mist in You recipe on page 158.)

Advice from a Stylist

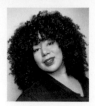

Nina Woodley, owner of Pure Avidity Salon in Orlando, FL

As the child of a Mexican mother and an African American father, I always felt different. Pretty much from the day I was born, people made comments about my hair, which was extremely dry, big, and frizzy. It was like wool! When I was a toddler, my mom's friend taught her how to do braids, cornrows, and box braids with beads. That became our way of "controlling" my curls, but with enough hair for three people, it could take seven to nine hours to do it. In kindergarten, one of our neighbor's kids threw handfuls of sand at my braided hair while we were playing at the park. When I came home, my mother was really upset. I had never seen her react like that regarding my hair. It made me realize that it really was different— and not in a good way.

I relaxed my hair until I was twenty-eight years old. But the summer after I finished cosmetology school, I decided I didn't want to chemically straighten it anymore. And I've never looked back. It took about eighteen months to grow out my relaxer, and in the process, I also grew. I was okay with the maintenance and time it required because it was authentically me! My hair became healthier, and people with similar hair started seeking my professional advice. This led me to become a curl specialist, which was a game changer for me! As a hairstylist, I am able to help people, not by giving them a great blowout for a day but by showing them how to care for their naturally curly hair. This encourages their confidence and builds their self-esteem. This journey of learning to love my curls has led me to where I am today. My hair is still big and everywhere and sometimes a little frizzy, but I wouldn't have it any other way.

HOW TO LOVINGLY BUT FIRMLY APPROACH A CHILD WHO IS GOING THROUGH AN I-HATE-MY-CURLS PHASE

Childhood is full of things we have to learn to accept, and that's not always easy. This includes your natural hair texture. There comes a time in grade school or middle school when many curlies insist on straightening and flat-ironing their hair. A lot of it is cultural and social. Perhaps your child's friends or siblings have naturally straight hair or are addicted to their flat irons. Since kids usually long to fit in rather than stand out, your child may truly dislike what nature gave her. Another culprit may be naturally curly adults in her life who are hiding behind their own blown-out strands, and your child is just trying to mimic them. What to do?

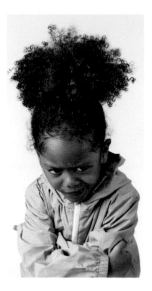

- Never talk badly about yourself in front of your child or to yourself. Our kids pick up on what we say and do and often copy it. Constantly putting down your own looks can affect your children. If you can't find positivity in your own hair, maybe it's time to try going outside your comfort zone to accept and embrace *your* natural texture too. This kind of healthy self-love will be contagious.

- Find curly hair role models for your child to talk to for inspiration and ask them their secrets for curl-love. This can be via social media or in person. I've had plenty of people stop me in the grocery store to ask about my hair, and I don't mind at all—in fact, I love it! You can also seek out friends and family members who have healthy relationships with their hair. In particular, curl-loving teens and young adults can encourage your children to love what nature gave them.

- Help your children manage their hair. This is especially important if their hair changes during puberty, which happens often. Books and curl specialists can provide tips and insight. Just be gentle in how you suggest these resources. You don't want to accidentally send the message that their hair or anything about their appearance is not okay or needs to be fixed.

- If your child has seen kiosks with flat irons at the mall, have a conversation about them. The salespeople tend to clack these devices at anyone with wavy or curly hair, promising that the flat iron will change their lives, all the while sending the message that they can't possibly be happy with the strands they have. Bring up the possibility that salespeople are trying to make curlies feel inferior just so they can sell products. Everyone has to make a living—but it shouldn't include making people feel bad about their hair.

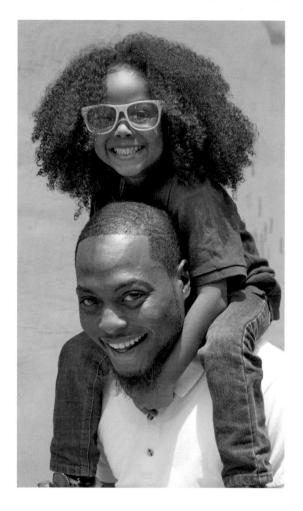

- Spa birthday parties are popular with young girls, and it's not always easy for your child to skip a blowout if her friends are getting them. This was always a dilemma when my daughter, Shey, was invited to these events. I felt that this reinforced that young girls should blow out their curls. I would tell Shey just to have her hair braided with her natural texture, but of course she got a blow-fry. You don't have to make everything into a curly power issue, but mention that she can say "no" to a blowout and still have fun.

Curly Kid Inspiration

Lindsay Olmo

I've always really liked my curly hair. Because almost everyone in my family, from my dad to my aunts to my cousins, had curls, it was just normal to me. I was also lucky to have a hair guru in my aunt. She would send me different hair products and give me curly tips and eventually led me to a stylist who knew curls.

When I was pregnant, I'd rub my belly and say, "Healthy and curly. Healthy and curly," because I had no idea how to take care of a kid with straight hair. Luckily, my wishes came true with my daughter *and*

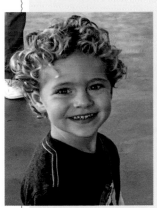

my son. It's almost embarrassing how many compliments my eight-year-old daughter, Ella, gets on her hair. When she was little, we couldn't go to a store or restaurant without masses of people coming up

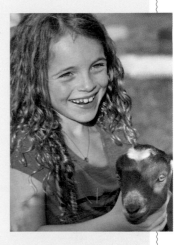

to us and asking me what I did to her hair. Now that she's older, people come up to her all the time. She's very shy, but she's used to it. My son, Aden, also loves his curls, and when I cut them recently, he let me know he was not pleased that I had "taken off his curls."

Since they were newborns, I've never used shampoo or any products with sulfates and mostly have washed their hair with conditioner. As a result, their curls are super-healthy, and even though they're very active, they never get knots. My kids know not to play with their hair while it's drying, that brushes and combs are just for dolls, and that we don't use towels on our hair. Since curly hair care has been part of their lives from the beginning, it's second nature to my kids, and so is loving their hair.

• I know many curly girls and guys who have taken their favorite products to the home of a friend who has a young curly-in-waiting. There, they give a curl-love class without expecting anything in return except seeing that little girl's face light up when she sees her true curl potential for the first time.

• Curly girls and guys who have embraced their hair love to share information and advice about their newfound hair freedom. I cannot tell you how many times I have heard stories of one curly giving verbal tutorials on the street to total strangers (while her friends or family members wait patiently). One woman told me she actually printed up small cards with her tips—like never use a brush and wash with conditioner—because she got asked about her hair so often and it was

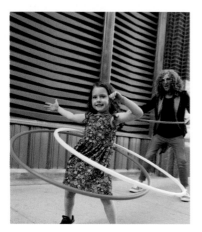

easier than scrounging for a pen and paper on a street corner. So why not host a party or sleepover where you can invite a curl scout or self-educated curl friend to come and give a CG Method tutorial and talk about embracing what nature gave you? Invite all your friends who straighten their hair (including those who don't admit it) and curl it forward. For a kids' sleepover, even naturally straight-haired friends can learn about good hair care and the glory of natural hair.

TALKING TO YOUR ASPIRING UNDERAGE STYLIST

One of my dear clients, Jamie, came home from work one day to a trail of perfect blond spiral curls leading to her youngest daughter's room. Her eight-year-old daughter had decided to cut off her four-year-old sister's curls. A wave of nausea swept over Jamie. After the shock faded, she learned that her older daughter was sick of all the positive attention her younger sister's beautiful curls were getting.

Curly Kid Inspiration

Claire Birkett

On the whole, my daughter Serenna loves her hair. She thinks it's incredible that her hair is long and straight when it's wet but short and curly when it's dry! We have been using the CG Method since she was so young that she just accepts it and allows the washing, scalp massage, and leave-in conditioner. And she loves her silk pillowcase.

We try very hard to boost Serenna's image of her hair by saying how special she is to have curls. However, this is hard when there aren't a lot of curly role models and there's only one curly Disney princess. So we try to find books and films that have curly characters.

We have taught Serenna how to manage the attention she receives for her hair. We're often asked, "Is that her natural hair?" along with references to Shirley Temple. That hasn't always been easy, particularly when people don't know their own boundaries and try to touch her hair. Luckily, she's a confident child and when complimented, will usually say, "Thank you!"

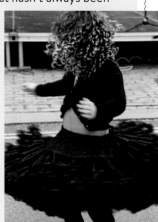

"Clearly, she was trying to get my attention, so I tried not to react with anger even though I was distraught," Jamie told me. If this happens to you, or your child cuts her own hair, explain that you don't like what she's done and that there will be consequences for her behavior. Let her know that you will put away the scissors and that she will be supervised when she wants to use them. If all signs point to her exercising the need to express herself artistically, offer better ways to be creative. Get a doll or mannequin head and a spray bottle filled with water so she can play with the hair and pretend to be a stylist. Then kindly but firmly remind your budding little stylist that only a hairdresser or other adult is allowed to cut any family member's hair.

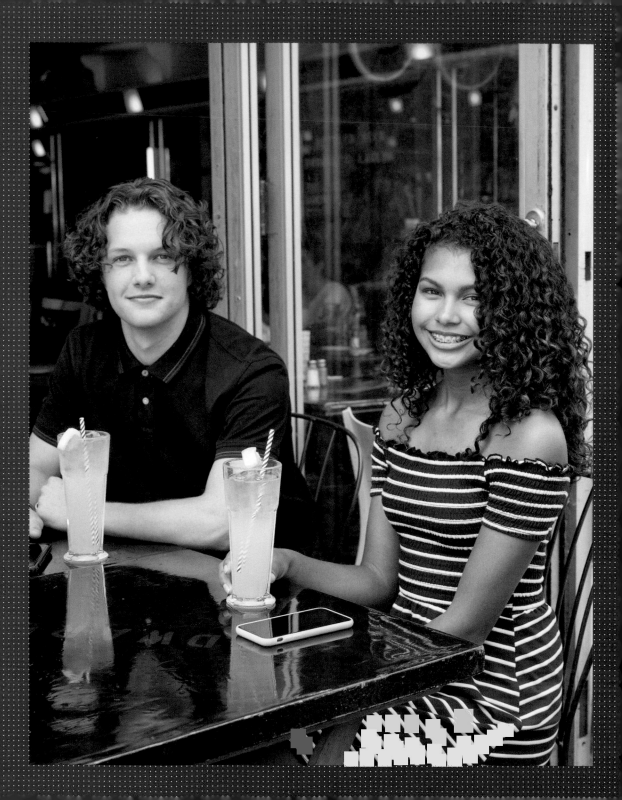

Four

The Tween & Teen Years

There are no bad curls, just misunderstood curls.

~~~~~~~~~~~~~~

I f you're between the ages of about 10 and 18, I don't need to tell *you* that this time in your life is filled with lots of changes. Your body. Your skin. And possibly your hair. Maybe it was wavy in grade school and has turned curly, or your curls have become tighter. Hair can also get oilier or drier. (Thank you, hormones!) The good news is that you're reading this book. And once you learn how to care for your hair—both what to do and what *not* to do—you'll see how simple it can be to work with your curls and, as a result, make them something you actually love. I've seen it happen over and over and over again: Curlies who thought they had "bad curls" or didn't like their hair and longed for a friend's silky, straight strands learned how to give their hair the right TLC and discovered gorgeous waves, curls, and coils. Now it's *their* hair that is the envy of friends and stops strangers on the street. My point is that your hair-care actions *can* make a difference in the outcome. Just give the CG Method a try, and with a little time you'll see that gorgeous hair has always been on top of your head. It was just hiding.

The CG Method for Tweens and Teens

- Stand under the running shower water until your hair is thoroughly wet. Resist the urge to touch your hair with your hands and just let the water cascade through your curls.

- Apply silicone- and sulfate-free conditioner to the pads of your fingers on one hand, and rub your hands together so it gets onto the pads of the other.

- The amount of conditioner you use depends on the length and thickness of your hair, so it may take some time to figure out. Generally, the tighter or drier the curl, the more you need to hydrate and detangle. Also, you will probably need less as your hair gets healthier.

- Splay your fingers and place them directly on your scalp.

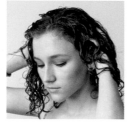

- Gently massage your scalp from the crown of your head to the nape of your neck. Be firm but gentle. Too much motion can cause frizz, knots, and tangles.

- Starting on one side of your head, very gently let your fingers glide downward

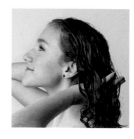

through small sections of your curls. This helps you carefully untangle knots, remove loose strands that have accumulated, and organize the curls into their natural position. Avoid using a comb or brush.

- We can lose 100 to 125 hairs per day, so don't be surprised if you have a bunch of loose hairs in your hands after gliding your fingers through your wet curls. Just take note of it so you know what is a normal amount for you.

- Avoid forcefully pulling at knots and tangles. Instead, just apply more conditioner to those areas. Got a serious knot that you can't see? Try to gently untangle it while looking in the mirror or ask someone else to help so that you'll avoid accidentally tearing your hair.

- If you have long hair, scrunch small sections up toward the scalp, because the action of finger-combing through longer hair can make curls stretch out. Scrunching reminds your curls of their natural shape.

- Stand out of the way of the running water. Cup your hands together under the water and toss it over small sections of hair to rinse out the conditioner. (I call this "the baptism.") Standing directly under the running water can rinse too much conditioner from your hair; the baptism gives you more control. Deciding whether to rinse out all the conditioner or just some of it takes some trial and error as you see how your hair looks best. You can rinse out most or all of it if you have waves or loose curls and leave more in for coarser, tighter curls since they tend to be drier and more frizz-prone. (Some people with really tight curls often don't need to rinse out any conditioner.) That may sound strange since we're so used to rinsing our hair thoroughly, but curly hair needs the extra moisture to remain hydrated and frizz-free. You may worry that leaving conditioner in will make your hair greasy, but that word is almost never part of a curly girl's or guy's vocabulary, and it won't make it crunchy, hard, or sticky when you're using products that don't contain sulfates and silicone.

- *Squeeze-quench* is a term I use to describe the process of using your hands to squeeze small sections of your hair in an upward motion toward the scalp. This will encourage your natural curl formation. The best way to do it is to bend over at the waist. If you hear a luscious squishy sound, that means your mission of hydration has been accomplished. When you squeeze-

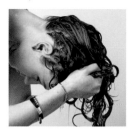

quench, a milky residue of excess water and conditioner may seep through your fingers. The hair naturally drinks up and absorbs the conditioner it needs to stay properly hydrated and usually drips and releases what it doesn't. Have a plastic container on hand to collect the milky residue. If you feel like your hair needs more conditioning, you can pour it back into your hair and rinse again or use it after you get out of the bath or shower and leave it in.

- A traditional terry-cloth towel has fibers that can ruffle the hair's cuticle, causing frizz and disturbing each curl's natural shape. With a traditional towel, you also can't feel the water content in the hair and how much water you want to remove or keep in. This also applies to microfiber towels. So once you're out of the bath or shower, use a paper towel, an old T-shirt, or multipurpose towels, which can be found at Home Depot or at office supply or other big-box stores, to gently squeeze small sections of the hair upward toward the scalp. This will remove excess water and encourage the curls' natural shape. If you want curls that are a bit looser or less defined, very gently blot small sections of hair from the scalp to the ends rather than scrunching it up.

A silicone- and alcohol-free gel can help define curls and reduce frizz. Simply pour a small amount into the palm of one hand, rub your hands together, and bend over at the waist. Lightly apply the gel to the landscape of the hair. You can also apply it to small sections by scrunching them up with gel in your hand. Again, the amount you use is determined through trial and error, but I'd start with a very small amount at first, because often less is more.

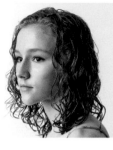

Try as hard as possible not to touch your curls as they dry. I know this isn't easy, but it will help prevent frizz and keep curls from separating. Also, be careful if you're getting dressed as your hair is drying, since pulling clothing over your head can mess up your curls too.

Long or thick hair can take a while to dry, so if you don't want to go to sleep or leave for school with damp hair, use a blow-dryer with a diffuser or a hooded helmet dryer (surprisingly inexpensive online).

If you use styling gel, your curls may feel like they're in what I call a product cast—a light film of gel surrounding each curl—once your hair is completely dry.

Keeping the hair in the gel cast is great if you have a special occasion later in the day or if it's raining. When it's party time or the weather improves—or if you want your curls to look more open—bend over at the waist and simply scrunch your hair upward to release the cast and curl. Then place your splayed fingers onto your scalp and gently shuffle them at the roots. Carefully remove your fingers from your hair, trying not to rake them through your curls. Then stand upright and, while looking at the ceiling, give your head one more shake.

You need to fully co-wash your hair only every two or three days. The rest of the time, you can just wet it in the shower or put it in a pineapple (see page 51) and let it dry. That said, if your hair looks great on your designated cleansing day, just leave it! Skip the co-wash and embrace your hair's natural beauty.

If your hair becomes noticeably oily, it could be from overwashing or using too much product—especially those that contain silicone. (See the section on products, starting on page 41, for other ingredients to avoid.) Oily hair can also mean that you're touching your curls too much, because oil from your hands gets onto your strands. This can also loosen the curl formation.

If you notice a strange odor, it could be from shampoo or conditioner residue building up on your scalp. This comes from using too much of these products, not massaging the scalp enough while cleansing, or not rinsing well. You do not need to wash your hair more often. You need to examine your cleansing method and adjust accordingly.

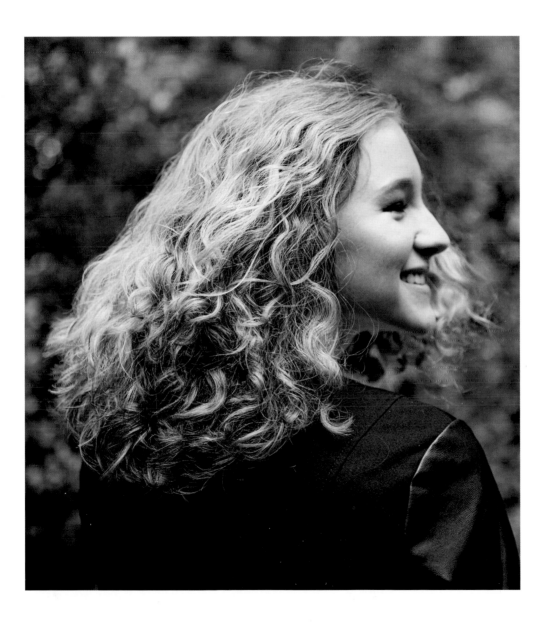

THE CURL IS MIGHTIER THAN THE FLAT IRON

You probably have many friends who own flat irons. Perhaps you own one too. But if you want to get the healthiest, most gorgeous curls possible, you must step away from the heat tools. Some flat irons and blow-dryers claim to be better for the hair than others and even brag about their "healthy" or "safe" plates. Sorry, that's just not true. Those words are pure marketing. Anything that is an *iron* and can get hot enough to smooth out even the tightest curls can cause damage and breakage and negatively alter your texture forever! Trust me, it's not pretty.

The truth is this: *Any* blow-dryer or flat iron, cheap or expensive, is not good for your hair. Have you ever seen an iron burn on clothing? You can never erase it. We never put a scalding hot iron on a cashmere sweater or delicate silk dress—so why do it to your hair, which is an organic fiber too? Now, you may think that you don't need to worry because you're young and so is your hair. But even occasional blowouts and flat-ironing can cause hair to burn, break off, and dry out, and too much heat-styling over the years can cause permanent damage to *any* hair, young, old, or in-between. On the other hand, air-drying (or using a diffuser when necessary) and never applying heat directly to your hair will leave it shiny, full, and gorgeous.

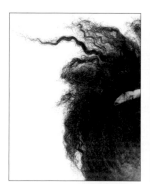 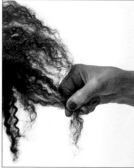

Even occasional blowouts and flat-ironing cause hair to burn and break.

When my daughter, Shey, was in her early teens, her hair appeared straighter and straighter, and she had a halo of broken flyaways at the top of her head. I wasn't sure what was up. *Maybe it's puberty and hormones*, I thought. *Or maybe it's a change in the seasons*. When I asked Shey, she insisted it was because she was wearing her hair in a ponytail all the time. That made sense to me until one day I was putting her laundry away in her closet and stumbled upon what I had suspected but couldn't believe: a flat iron! I was shocked, dumbfounded, and bewildered. For a natural-hair advocate like me, it might as well have been drugs that she was hiding! Not only did I know the damage that straightening her hair could do, but I was also upset that she didn't want to embrace who she was naturally.

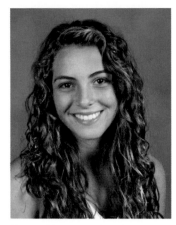

Shey and her natural curls

Around the same time, a friend of Shey's—let's call her Taylor—became totally hooked on flat-ironing her curls, which were truly amazing and beautiful. In her obsessed state, Taylor told me she could feel her hair crinkling back to coils in the middle of the night so she would often wake up to iron it out. Yes, she'd get up and out of bed to flatten her hair with heat! Even worse? Taylor was one of the best athletes in her school. But once she discovered flat ironing, she stopped breaking a sweat of any kind because it would cause her hair to curl up. In fact, Taylor and many of her friends actually brought their flat irons with them everywhere—school, sports, and part-time jobs—just in case any curl dared to escape the straitjacket.

But back to the moment I found the flat iron in Shey's room. You know the movie *Mommie Dearest*, where Joan Crawford screams, "No wire hangers ever!"? That was me, except I was screaming, "No flat irons ever!" Shey, who was downstairs with Taylor at the time, came running upstairs to see me holding the iron up to the heavens like a crazy person. She was stunned to see that she was busted.

"It's not mine," she said. "It's Taylor's."

"No, it's not," Taylor said, popping her head in the door.

This was literally *ironic* for anyone who knows me. It's the hair equivalent of bringing cooked meat into a vegetarian restaurant. But when I took a deep breath, I realized that I had to let Shey find her own wavy way. I had to let her make her own mistakes with her hair (and in life) or else she'd never learn. Thankfully, her flat iron phase was short-lived and now she loves and embraces her natural wavy texture. But I can't say the same for Taylor, who a decade later is still straightening her strands. The gorgeous thickness of her hair has decreased a lot. In fact, not much was left when I saw her recently, which made me sad, because I knew how beautiful and healthy her natural hair had been. Plus, I can't imagine how exhausting, it must be for her to maintain.

In life and with hair, we tend to want what we don't have, and often we prefer to fit in rather than stand out. I get it. I felt the same way when I was struggling with my curls as a teen. I think it's even harder today, when there are all these outside forces perpetually reinforcing totally flat, straight strands—unnaturally straight strands—not only in day-to-day life but also on social media and

SUNGLASSES AND HEADPHONES

Be careful and gentle when removing big headphones. Hair can get caught in them and rip or tear. Also be careful if you put your sunglasses on your head to hold your hair back. This can cause major breakage. Hair can easily get wrapped around the nose bar prongs and side hinges and can be very hard to remove without serious damage.

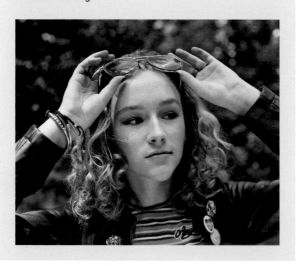

TV. Well, you should know that that hair is not real, whether it's on Instagram or the red carpet. Not only is it blown or flattened into submission, but it's also often filled in with hairpieces, extensions, or wigs, important details that these "reality" shows,

Perfect curls are not real. Real curls are not perfect.

celebrities, and beauty bloggers don't want to share. These aren't good options for anyone. Extensions tug on your real hair so it can break, fall out, and cause your hairline to recede. Unfortunately, once the hair recedes, it doesn't always grow back. Wigs worn regularly actually suffocate the hair and skin beneath it. The rare times when you *do* see curly or wavy celebrities, their hair is typically straightened *first* before being curled with a curling iron. My point is that being surrounded by these unattainable images makes you wonder why your curls don't look like that, and then you feel bad about your hair.

Often, just getting a haircut can make you hate your hair, since hairstylists often assume everyone wants their hair blown out after a cut, and there's a sense that you should be grateful to your stylist for doing so. Years ago at a hair convention, a hairdresser came over to me, leaned in, and whispered, "If you let me blow out your hair, you'll fall in love with me." *Um, I don't think so! Someone hold me back!*

Then there are the blowout bars that seem to be on every corner in every major city around the globe, ready and willing to take you out of your "misery." That is, until the next time, or until it rains. This sets you up for a hard-to-maintain, unsustainable straight-hair lifestyle and is tacitly telling you that you should spend a lot of time, money, and effort to hide your natural hair.

Sometimes the pressure to straighten comes from your own family. The stories I've heard over the years are astounding. Parents throwing money at their children, begging them to get their bountiful curls straightened or cut off! Others tell me how exhausted and disheartened they are by their friends', family's, or coworkers'

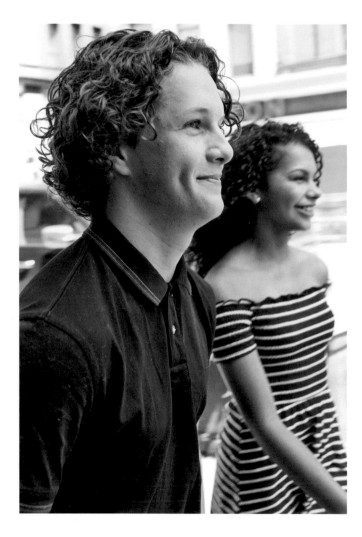

negative hair comments. I don't think these loved ones understand how much they are hurting their curly-haired friend or family member. My advice to them and to you if you have similar experiences: Tell your parents, partner, friends, colleagues, and anyone else, "I value the opinion that you keep to yourselves."

Even if you straighten your hair temporarily, it takes incredible time and effort to sustain. Plus, it means your life revolves around your hair. A sweaty workout or swim in the pool seems out of the question, and you find yourself watching the weather and fearing any humidity or rain. This means you're taking energy away from many other things—like actually living your life! But if you embrace your curls, waves, coils, or kinks and learn how to care for them—which is *a lot* easier and less time-consuming than straightening—you'll not only save time but also feel more comfortable in your own skin.

Curly Kid Inspiration

Grey Rozensweig

Hair is an extension of the self, and hair length is part of an ingrained supposition about gender. The way I wear my hair tells people who I am before I do, just like my clothes. If my hair is long, if my clothes are feminine, my gender is perceived as female. When my hair is short and my clothes are what is regarded as masculine, I am perceived as androgynous, or in some rare cases, male. *Passing* is a colloquial term used in the LGBTQ+ community to describe being perceived as the gender identity you more closely identify with. I think gender as a binary idea is dead. Wearing my hair short and my shirts buttoned up but still putting on rings and earrings is the way I best like to express myself—and the perception of the outside world

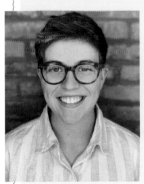

is important, but the joy of recognizing myself in the mirror is far greater than the fear of any ridicule surrounding my choices.

My hair has always been one of the easiest and most important ways in which I express myself. I felt stuck when it was long, always pulling it up to keep it out of my face or braiding it back. It felt out of place during the last few years I wore it long—but when I cut it short, the euphoria I felt when I looked in the mirror couldn't be achieved through any other physical change. New clothes, shoes—anything, really—couldn't compare with the way cutting my hair made me feel.

My absolute biggest advice, in no uncertain terms, is this: If you want to cut your hair, if you want to change it, do it! If you want to grow it long and paint your nails and be a boy, do it, do it, do it. The power of your curls is so amazing—expressing yourself through a hairstyle is incredibly fulfilling. Being able to look in the mirror and see the self you've always wanted to look like—*not* society's idea or expectation of you—is better than anything else.

HOW TO LOVE TEEN CURLS

TEACHING CURLS

When my daughter was fourteen years old, one of her friends started straightening her curly hair. It took an hour and a half, and she'd do it at 11:00 p.m. after finishing her homework. Then she'd try to sleep carefully so she wouldn't mess up her hard work. Despite this, she'd inevitably have to spend time doing a few touch-ups in the morning. One day I asked her why she straightened her hair when her curls were so beautiful.

"This boy I have a crush on said he liked it straight," she confided.

"If he really likes you, he'll like you straight *or* curly," I said. It was a small comment, but as a result, she put down her flat iron and spent the time cultivating her natural hair texture.

A couple of years later, she reminded me of that conversation and told me it had taught her a valuable lesson: Don't straighten your hair—or do *anything else* in life—because of what someone else thinks. Amen!

> ### PRODUCT INGREDIENTS
>
> It's fun to experiment with and test out new products for your skin, hair, and body. But you must read the ingredient lists and make sure the products don't contain the following: sulfates, sodium lauryl sulfate (S.L.S.), silicones, alcohol, parabens, and formaldehyde.

CLEANSING T-ZONE SCALPS AND DRY HAIR

It's possible to have dry hair and an oily scalp—often at the front, around the temples, and at the nape of the neck. This is especially the case if you have combination skin on your face—oily on the forehead, nose, and chin but dry on the cheeks. The oil on the scalp attracts dirt and bacteria that must be rinsed off regularly to keep the scalp healthy. But it's not necessary to remove *all* the oils from your scalp; in fact, it's not good for you. You need a fine layer of sebum—called the acid mantle—for protection. My solution is to give the scalp a gentle massage and a good water rinsing followed by conditioner or a spritz of lavender spray—no harsh detergent necessary! (See the recipes in Chapter 6.)

HOW TO BREAK THE HAIR-STRAIGHTENING HABIT

If you really want to break the straightening habit, congrats! You're making a life-changing decision, and your hair will thank you. It's *much* easier than having to grow out a chemical straightener (which can take a year or more), but it still requires some patience and practice. Start here:

- Begin to notice other teens with curls in the world around you—on the street, at the mall, at school, and so on. Notice what you do and don't like about their hair. Also, visit all the curly social media sites you can. Many are really inspiring and show you what you're striving for.

- Get rid of sulfate- and silicone-filled shampoo and other products, brushes, combs, blow-dryers, and flat irons. Replace them with products that are free of these chemicals and made for curly hair. Once you

NO PRODUCTS ON HAND?

Even if you don't have time or products, you can give your curls a refresh.

- Wet your hands in the sink.

- Bend forward at your waist and tilt your head forward. Scrunch your hair upward with your wet hands. This should reactivate any gel that's already in your hair.

- For more volume, place splayed fingers on your scalp and gently shuffle them. Flip your head upright and carefully remove your fingers from your hair so you don't disrupt any curls.

- If you have any fractured or dispersed curls, wet a finger, wind a curl around it, and hold it for a minute. Repeat this on any curls as needed. You will be amazed at how quickly they can spring back!

NATURAL HAIR COMES IN FIRST

It was so exciting when Connecticut's Kaliegh Garris won Miss Teen USA in 2019, because it had been twenty years since the pageant had crowned a winner with natural hair. (When you do see curls on young women in pageants, it's usually the result of a curling iron used on hair that's been blown straight first.) After winning, Kaliegh told *Elle* magazine, "When I was younger, I competed with extensions in my hair a lot, but over time I just got more heat damage, and my hair just kept getting shorter and shorter because it kept burning off. I had to stop worrying about where I fit in and have enough strong will within myself to be comfortable with who I am and embrace my natural hair. And that's one reason why I'll always compete with my natural hair." Although plenty of naysayers told Kaliegh she looked better with straight strands and should put in extensions for the pageant, she trusted herself. "I know what I look like with straight hair, with extensions, and with my curly hair, and I feel more confident and comfortable with my natural hair," she says. Now, that's a winner!

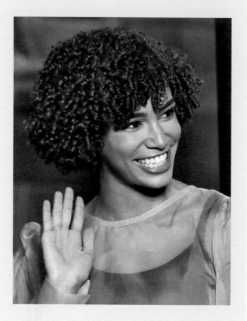

treat your curls with TLC by using more healthful products, your curls will look and feel better than ever. Try to avoid combs or brushes completely. If you must use one or the other, do so only when the hair is protected by conditioner.

• Initially, stick with your regularly scheduled cleansing program, simply swapping shampoo for sulfate-free cleanser or conditioner and allowing the hair to air-dry naturally or be diffused instead of using a brush and blow-frying. As you see your curls emerge, you will become more confident and begin to experiment with how often you should co-wash your hair.

- Once that happens, see if you can push it off just one more day and observe how your curls look with just a spot cleanse with What Knots? spray or refresh with Mist in You (see Chapter 6 for recipes.) You will be surprised to see the hidden beauty unfurling.

- While you allow the hair to air-dry, do your best not to touch or disturb the curls *at all.* Overtouching and fussing can equal frizz.

- You have to give your curls a chance. It may take a little while for you to accept them visually. Often this is the hardest part, because you are looking at a different silhouette. Your curls will not be at their full potential initially. You must be patient and take into consideration that the hair has to rehabilitate and regain its own curl consciousness. I can promise that if you are consistent in your approach and applications, your hair will improve *every single day.* Curls are very forgiving when treated right.

- Some people are tempted to fall off the curl wagon and consider straightening their hair for "special occasions." But ask yourself this: What is so special about looking like everyone else? Straightening your curls occasionally is *not* okay. It's like smoking cigarettes every once in a while; you'd be surprised how much damage that "one time" or "every once in a while" can do. Most heat tools get to such high temperatures that they can bake cookies. In other words, singed hair is singed hair. Also, if you have been treating your curls well for a while and then go and strip them with the occasional shampoo and

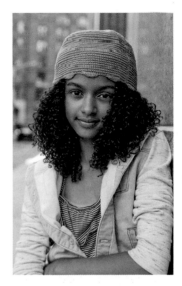

blow-fry, it will set you back. You'll dry out your hair and fray the ends, and it may take the curls a while to regain their shape. On the other hand, once you start to respect what your hair *is* rather than what it is not, you may never want to knowingly harm it again and you *will* see all your effort and curl-love care pay off. The curls will regain their shape, the frizz will disappear, and your curls will grow in healthier than ever. You'll be on curl autopilot and become a point of inspiration for other curlies.

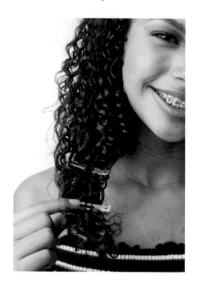

CLIPS TO LENGTHEN HAIR

Clips can help lengthen hair and tight curls while they dry or coax out curls that hide by the nape of the neck. When hair is wet, gently place a clip at the end of

HAIR-PULLING DISORDER

Trichotillomania, also called hair-pulling disorder, is a treatable condition that can affect people of any age. However, it typically develops somewhere during the tween and teen years. Those who suffer from this chronic condition have an uncontrollable urge to repeatedly pull their own hair out from their scalp, eyebrows, eyelashes, or pubic area. For many, this pulling can be a way to deal with stress, anxiety, tension, and frustration. Unfortunately, the result can be bald spots and shortened or thinning hairs, which in and of themselves can make you feel even more anxious and stressed—especially if those hairs don't grow back. Some people pull the hair while focused on something else, like watching TV or reading, or when they're bored. Risk factors include a family history of the disorder; having other conditions like anxiety, depression, or obsessive-compulsive disorder; and experiencing very stressful situations. There are psychologists and other experts who specialize in trichotillomania treatment.

each curl so that gravity pulls on it and adds weight, helping to naturally stretch it out. When hair is dry, use care removing clips as hair can wrap around them as it dries.

GIVING CURLS A LIFT

If you've got really loose waves that tend to fall flat during the day, here are two tips:

- Conditioner may weigh the hair down if you apply too much. Try leaving it on for less time and rinsing it out completely.

- You can give hair a lift by placing a yoga mat on the floor and putting a towel over it. Gently rub a moderate amount of gel into your hair and lie down on your back on the mat. Spread your damp, gelled locks around your head like a veil. Use a hair dryer with a diffuser to dry your hair. Because the hair is resting on the floor, not being pulled down from the roots by gravity, its weightlessness guarantees body and bounce without frizz.

THINKING OF CHEMICALLY STRAIGHTENING YOUR HAIR? HERE'S WHY YOU SHOULD THINK AGAIN.

Chemical straightening may *seem* like an answer to your prayers, but there are plenty of downsides.

- Very strong chemicals are required to change the bonds in the hair from curly to straight. You and the stylist may require masks to limit inhalation. The chemicals are so harsh that they can cause damage like split ends or breakage at the roots, leaving a halo of hair floating above your part.

- These treatments can take a lot of time—anywhere from four to six hours at a salon—and you have to repeat them every four to six months. This is the case even when you're just getting your curly roots touched up, because the rest of the hair needs to be covered with special protective products.

- They can also be super-expensive, anywhere from $200 to $1,000 per treatment.

- Blow-drying is required to keep hair straight, causing more damage.

- The only way chemically straightened hair can go back to curly is to wait for your hair to grow out, and that can take months or years.

- Chemically straightened hair does not necessarily even look good! Over time, it usually looks dull, worn-out, and frizzy.

GO STRAIGHT TO CURLS

If you have already tried chemical straightening and want to go back to curly, that's great! It will take time, patience, and willpower, but it will pay off big-time—because you'll love the hair that's revealed at the end of the journey.

- As soon as you decide to go back to curly, stop using cleansers containing sulfates and silicone ASAP. These harsh detergents can dry out hair that's already thirsty and damaged from chemical treatments.

- Hydrate your hair with daily conditioning treatments ASAP too, to repair the damage from harsh straightening chemicals. This helps you make sure the new curly growth is its healthiest. Some curlies I've worked with say that seeing any frizz as their curls grow in is enough to send them right back to chemical straightening. But that halo is just hair that hasn't been hydrated enough. Keep up your dedication to going curly by using conditioner, conditioner, and more conditioner.

- No more brushes. The act of brushing or combing the hair actually pulls it out from the root and interferes with your curls' formation, causing fused and dispersed curls. Even when your hair is more straight than curly, you should kick

BACKPACKS, BAG STRAPS, AND CURLS

It's easy for long curls to get trapped under the strap of your backpack or any shoulder bag.

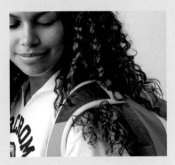

Unfortunately, when we realize this, we unconsciously yank the trapped hair out from beneath the straps, tearing and fracturing the curls. Do this a few times a day every day for weeks and months, and it will make one side of the hair appear stringy and weaker. The solution is simple: Move your hair off your shoulder before slinging on your bag. And if hair does get stuck under the strap, which it will, first lift the bag off your shoulder and *then* move the hair, rather than pulling the hair out from underneath it.

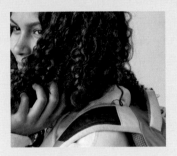

the brushing habit. Instead, use your fingers to comb through the hair and do so *only* while it's wet and drenched with conditioner.

- As the healthy new curls sprout, they act as little springboards and push out the straightened hair. The result is regrowth of your natural, curly texture at the top and your chemically straightened hair at the bottom. Sticking with this in-between phase is the most challenging part. Just keep the final goal in mind. If needed, find pictures of gorgeous curls you love and put them where you can keep your eyes on the prize.

- Get your hair trimmed often. Most curly girls don't want to cut off all their straight hair, but you need regular trims to oxygenate the ends, which helps hair grow.

CURL LOVE IS FOREVER

There are three basic things to remember in order to love your curls for life.

1. Your hair is like a living garden that accompanies you wherever you go.

2. Conditioner is to the hair what water is to the body. This and TLC are necessities that your curls can't live without.

3. Give your hair oxygen by trimming the ends. When you prune a plant, you're helping it take oxygen and water from the atmosphere. Apply this thinking to the ends of your own hair and you will be amazed at what a difference a little trim will do!

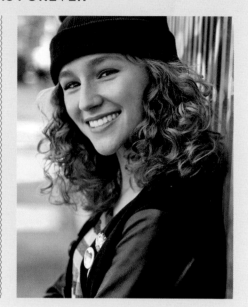

- Experiment with ways to style your hair while you're growing it out. Use leave-in conditioner and slick your hair back in a classic knot at the back of the head or off to the side. Also, try other updos, bandannas, and hats. Just make sure you don't pull your hair back too tightly or you'll cause the hairline to recede. Also, look for fabric-covered ponytail holders, not those with clasps, which can cut through the hair like a saw when your head moves.

- Never use curling irons or, even worse, perm the straightened ends to match your curly roots. The hair can break off, which will further damage already dried-out straight hair. Setbacks set you back!

- Don't blow-fry and flat-iron roots to match the straight ends. The new roots are healthy, unprocessed hair, and heat-styling will disrupt their natural curl formation.

• Eat a healthy diet that helps hair grow. That includes leafy green vegetables and natural proteins.

• When you freak out and want to reach for that blow-dryer and flat iron, remember that straightening your curls is temporary, lasting only until it rains or your next shower. Loving and living with your curls is easy and natural. Plus, over time, all those chemicals and heat will leave you with unhealthy, damaged, lifeless hair that requires even more time and energy. Nurture your curls and you'll eventually have gorgeous, healthy strands without much effort. Just visualize how your curly hair will look in a few months to help you keep going.

PRECONDITIONING FOR HEALTHY CURLS

This is perfect for long, thick curls and for those that have become water-resistant, or hydrophobic, something that happens to very thick, dense, curly hair. Water beads up on the hair a little like water on duck feathers. The problem is that if water doesn't get the hair wet enough, it will not absorb the conditioner applied, starving the hair of true hydration.

• Apply a silicone- and sulfate-free conditioner to dry hair, making sure all curls are covered. If needed, add more directly to any knotted areas. Leave this on for at least ten minutes and up to an hour before bath or shower time. This preconditions the hair, which allows it to absorb the conditioner and water more quickly.

SEASONS OF HAIR

The skin renews itself constantly, typically every thirty days, but the hair does not, so treat it right! In the summer, hair grows more quickly than it does in winter. It's also believed to grow more slowly at night than during the day.

- If you're worried about drips, put on a shower cap. However, when conditioner alone is applied to dry hair, it usually won't drip, because your thirsty hair will soak it up.

- While you are waiting, periodically use a spray bottle containing warm water to spritz over the hair. Try not to let the conditioner dry out. Spritzing helps reinforce and push the conditioner deep into the hair, softening any knots.

- Get into the bath or shower and wet the hair.

- You may notice how quickly the hair absorbs the water as opposed to repelling it, which can happen if hair is dry when you usually get in the shower. FYI, if at times when you *don't* precondition, your hair feels like it's repelling water even when you stand under the shower stream for a while, check your products. Chances are they contain synthetic oils and silicone. If they do, stop using them ASAP. Oil and water don't mix.

- Continue cleansing, conditioning, detangling, and organizing your curls with the CG Method.

KEEPING STRANDS HEALTHY DURING HARSH TIMES

I do not endorse tar shampoos, which are often recommended for dandruff, but if you insist on using them, you must at least protect your hair. Try this proactive approach.

1. Wet your hair and apply a silicone- and sulfate-free conditioner to the outermost layer, avoiding the roots. Let it sink in.

2. Apply the tar product to your fingertips and massage it in *only* at the scalp, avoiding the rest of the hair.

3. Rinse out the tar shampoo well with warm water. Water that is too hot dries the scalp even more. As the tar is rinsed away, it inevitably runs through the hair strands, so the conditioner acts as a protective barrier from the shampoo's harsh stripping effects. This really makes a huge difference!

DANDRUFF AND ITS VICIOUS CYCLE

To paraphrase Albert Einstein, you cannot solve a problem in the same way you created it. This is true of most things, especially dandruff, something I have always believed is simply a dry scalp begging for moisture and friction. A common solution for people who think they have dandruff is to shampoo, often because it's the only time they feel a temporary relief from the chronic itchiness and inflammation. Also, some products claim that *not* shampooing enough can cause a buildup of oil and dead skin cells, leading to dandruff—but there is little evidence to support this. In reality, ingredients like the sodium in sulfates can strip oil from the scalp, leaving it dry, scaly, red, and itchy, or exacerbate the itchiness of a scalp that is already irritated. Other common shampoo components like silicone and the chemicals in fragrance just make matters worse.

But it's not just traditional shampoo that's the issue. Dandruff sufferers often cleanse with products that contain harsh ingredients like tar and other medically advised chemicals, which in and of themselves are extremely drying for skin and hair. When you dehydrate the scalp, the result is more irritation, itchiness, and white flakes. These ingredients also leave your poor hair fibers parched and thirsty, so they don't look their best. In my opinion, this is like pouring gasoline on a fire that you're trying to put out. The problem is that often dandruff sufferers have been living with their symptoms and this self-inflicted cycle for so long that it's become "normal" to them. They are simply doing this by default: It's what they've always done and what dandruff-shampoo manufacturers tell us to do. Why would they know any better?

Curly Kid Inspiration

Shoshana Maisel

I remember being in elementary school, sitting at my desk during class, staring at the perfectly shiny and stick-straight hair of the girl who sat in front of me. Then I'd look down at my own frizzy mess and think, *It's just not fair!* I equated having straight hair with being beautiful, and the only time I felt pretty was when I straightened my hair. But that lasted only until it curled up again. Most of my friends had straight hair, and I was always envious of how easy it was for them to take care of their hair. It was almost no work at all! On the other hand, for me it was a full-time job.

The turning point was when I was twelve years old and a friend recommended a curly hair salon. It was the answer to my prayers. I remember looking in the mirror after my first experience at the curly salon and doing a double take. I couldn't believe it was me in the mirror. I couldn't believe that the same curls I had resented and despised so much throughout my entire life were . . . beautiful. Soon thereafter, my curls went from being

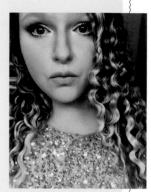

one of my biggest insecurities to my best friend. My hair gives me confidence every day.

I started cutting my own curls as soon as I learned how from *Curly Girl: The Handbook*. This opened a whole new world for me. Getting my hair cut used to be one of the things I dreaded most when I was younger. The hairdresser would always comment as she attempted to brush through my thick curls, muttering something under her breath that made me feel guilty and embarrassed. Plus, it always hurt! All of the unnecessary pulling and tugging usually resulted in a flood of tears. It's been almost nine years since I've gone to a hairdresser, and I'm proud to say it! I cut my own curls on a regular basis. It is quick, easy, and painless!

Today, strangers often stop to ask me about my hair. Being told that my hair is beautiful by strangers really makes my day, every single time. Embracing my curls made me finally feel beautiful.

When I was on my *Silver Hair* book tour, I was talking about the downside of using traditional shampoo. A woman in the audience raised her hand. "But I have to use special shampoo because I have dandruff," she said.

"Do you still have dandruff?" I asked.

"Yes. I've had it for years," she said. Years? Clearly this shampoo cycle wasn't working if she still had symptoms and hadn't experienced healing. Sidney Baker, MD, a preventive medicine specialist, once said, "If you are sitting on a tack, the answer is not to treat the pain. The solution is to find the tack and remove it." The same goes for your dandruff. The solution is not to just treat the symptoms— such as flakes—but to get to the root of the problem. Countless people can attest that they have been truly relieved from their dandruff once they stopped using detergent- and sulfate-filled shampoos.

PRODUCT OVERLOAD

The average woman slathers on an estimated twelve to twenty beauty and hair products a day! I'm not surprised by this number. I often see clients whose hair is laden with so much product that it is limp, lackluster, and unhealthy, and their scalp has flakes from product residue and dead skin cells. This overuse is on overload, and consumers of these products are becoming younger and younger, because manufacturers are targeting tweens and teens. Recently, I was looking at a friend's high school yearbook from the late 1980s. At first, I was struck by how unmanicured

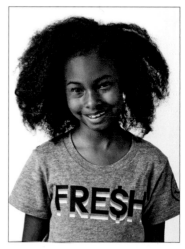

Too much bad product can lead to buildup and block hydration, drying out hair.

yet naturally healthy the teenagers looked. But then I remembered that this was actually *normal*. Piling on the products isn't surprising in our "more is more" society. But it's time to rethink this, not only to save time and money and avoid potential health risks, but also because we don't need all those gels, creams, lotions, potions, and cosmetics. We also don't need to try to erase, hide, or mask everything, from our natural smell to spots on our faces to kinks in our hair. I'm only half joking when I say that our great-grandchildren will have to go to portrait museums to see what a naturally aging woman used to look like.

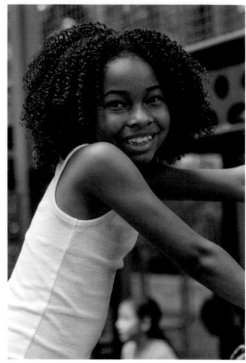

When the right amount of the best product is used, curls come alive.

YET ANOTHER REASON NATURAL IS BEST

A study conducted at the Silent Spring Institute in Newton, Massachusetts, analyzed eighteen different hair products, including hot oil treatments, anti-frizz hair polishers, leave-in conditioners, and relaxers. Results revealed that these products contained a total of forty-five endocrine disruptors. These are substances that disrupt hormones in our bodies, which can cause early puberty and an increased risk of hormone-related health issues such as uterine fibroids, infertility, and preterm births. Each product tested had between four and thirty of these ingredients, and eleven of them contained chemicals that are prohibited in the European Union or regulated under California's Proposition 65.

YOU ARE WHAT YOU EAT—AND SO ARE YOUR CURLS

When you eat healthy foods, your body and mind benefit—and so does your hair. "The look and feel of your curls is connected to what you put in your mouth. Certain nutrients not only help your body feel and function better, but they're also important for that shiny, bouncy hair you want," explains Esther Blum, MS, RD, CDN, CNS, integrative dietitian, and author of *Eat, Drink, and Be Gorgeous: A Nutritionist's Guide to Living Well While Living It Up.* "Since hair is 97 percent protein, you need this nutrient to help it grow and stay healthy." Eating healthy fats is also important, because they enhance the hair's natural oils, which leave it looking lush, shiny, and thick, not dull and lifeless, and help hydrate the scalp. These include omega-3 essential fatty acids, which can be found in salmon (preferably wild Alaskan), herring, anchovies, sardines, flaxseeds, and walnuts. It's also important to eat plenty of high-quality fats like avocado, avocado oil, coconut oil, olives, and olive oil. Getting enough iron—

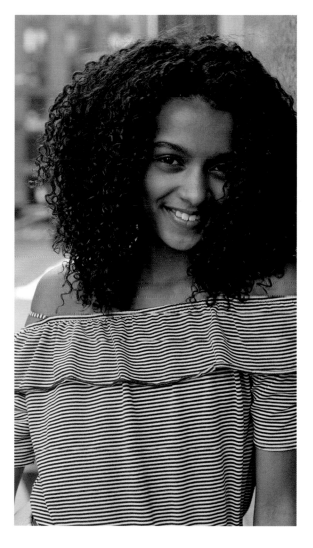

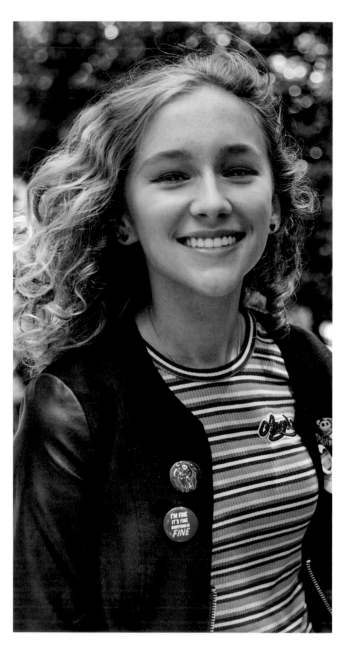

plentiful in foods like beef, liver, dark-meat turkey, eggs, and beans—and hyaluronic acid, found in bone broth, keeps hair from thinning. "Trace minerals like zinc, magnesium, and selenium may help thinning hair or hair loss," adds Blum. Find them in nuts like almonds, hazelnuts, walnuts, and cashews; seeds like pumpkin seeds; and whole grains like brown rice and steel-cut oats.

This is the best time (because it's now!) to really get to know your curls for their true selves. Meet your curls, be kind to them, nourish them, and you'll be friends forever. I promise.

Curly Kid Inspiration

Abby Cohen

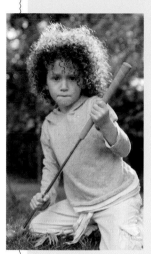

When I was younger, people told me over and over how unique my curls were and how lucky I was because "people spend so much money" to get hair like mine. Of course, these are compliments, but when you are eight years old and all the people telling you these things are adults, it does not mean anything. Being different is even harder when people are constantly telling you how cool or beautiful your hair is.

I felt left out because my hair could not do what other girls' hair could. I threw fits all the time in my bathroom because I was always so frustrated. For the majority of elementary school and middle school, I wore my hair in a ponytail. Needless to say, it took a really long time for me to love my curls, which was when I was around fifteen years old. A key factor in learning how to love my curls was finding the right products. I have tried probably every curly hair product out there and have finally found a combination that works and makes me feel confident.

Today, I do not mind that doing my hair the way I like takes a little more time, because it is worth it. It's a process to love your curls, and there is no secret formula (besides finding the right hair products). Now that I am nineteen, I know that having curly hair is a gift and it makes me stand out. And now it is important to me that I *do* stand out. No part of me wants to be just like everyone else or "normal."

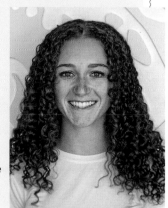

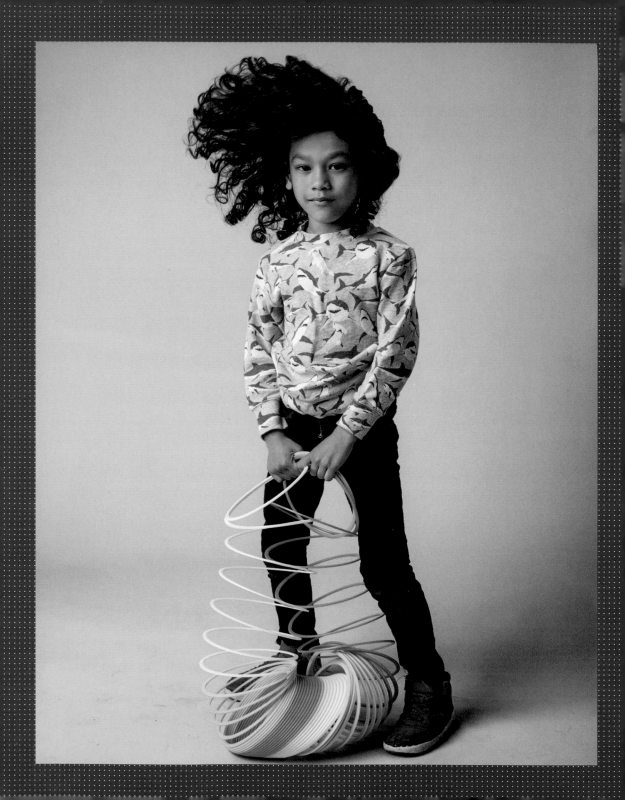

Five

Sporty Kids & Curly Hairstyles

Your hair is a part of you—not apart from you.

Sports and other physical activities are important for your child's health and well-being, and the lessons learned from being part of a team are priceless. But active curly kids need to give their hair some extra attention so that it doesn't get in their way while they're breaking a sweat and to prevent damage, split ends, and dryness. Of course, looking stylish while playing sports is important too!

Ponytails are the most common sporty style. A ponytail keeps hair out of your child's face and can look cute too. But the key factors to be aware of are how tightly it is pulled and the kind of elastic used to tie it back. When hair is pulled too tightly for too long, a disorder called traction alopecia can result. This is when the hairs fall out or become sparse, causing a receding hairline. You often see this with too-tight cornrows or braids as well. In some cases, these hairs won't grow back. Another issue is sunburn if the gaps between the tightly pulled braids are so wide that the skin is exposed. Keep ponytails as loose as you can. If they need to be tight, remove them immediately after the activity to reduce the amount of time the hair is pulled. If possible, use a soft, fabric-covered ponytail holder rather than an elastic band, which can saw at the hair and cause breakage as your child runs around. If an elastic band is a must, look for those without any metal.

CURLY HAIR WITH HOODS, HATS, SCARVES, AND MORE

When it comes to curlies, a little prep is needed before slipping on a hat, hood, wig, earmuffs, scarf, or other head covering. The hair should be positioned correctly beforehand to avoid flat, matted curls and to reduce frizz. Here's how:

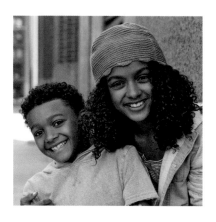

• Keep using the CG Method. Healthy, well-hydrated curls provide more cushioning and will revive more quickly once your child takes off her hat.

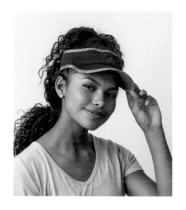

• Before putting on your child's hat or other head covering, apply gel directly to a clip or bobby pin. Pull up a clip-sized section of hair at the crown of the head, and place the clip or pin at the roots of the hair perpendicular to the scalp. You may need to use several clips. This keeps the roots elevated while the weight of what you're covering the hair with is pressing down on them.

- If the hair is longer than shoulder length, gently gather it at the nape of the neck with a fabric-covered ponytail holder. Twist the curly tail upward and anchor it to the back of the head with bobby pins.

- If your child has short curls around the front, take sections and twist them backward toward the crown. This keeps curls from getting disfigured and will regenerate movement when you set them free again.

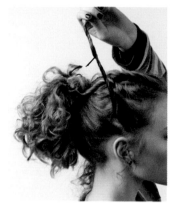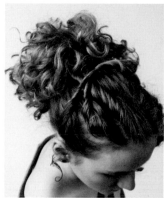

- After taking off your child's hat or other head covering, spritz the hair with lavender spray or wet your hands slightly with water. Have your child tilt her head to one side, place your damp fingers at the roots, and gently shuffle your fingertips to open the hair. Lift your hands off the scalp without running your fingers through the hair. Then scrunch upward the same way you scrunch gel into the hair while styling. Repeat on the other side.

- If your child wears a helmet and you want to give the top layer of hair more lift, lightly spritz a few of the flattened curls with lavender spray or water. Twist each section around your index finger, then slide the curl off and either pin or hold it in place with your fingers for a couple of minutes. (If water isn't available, just lick your finger to create an old-fashioned spit curl.)

SWIMMING WITH CURLS

The chlorine in pool water can dehydrate hair, give blond hair a green cast, and make brown hair look ashen. Salt water can also leave hair dry. These tips will help prevent these issues.

• Soak your child's Lycra swim cap in conditioner for a few minutes before she wears it. This protects the hair from the first gush of chlorinated water. If you don't have time to soak the cap, just rub the lining with conditioner.

• Before applying the swim cap, put conditioner in your hands, rub them together, and apply it in a downward motion to the top layer of your child's hair. This is even more important to do if your child doesn't have a swim cap.

• *Never* use sulfate-filled shampoo to wash hair after swimming. The combination of chlorine and sulfates adds a double dose of chemicals to the hair's delicate surface. And don't be fooled by products that promote themselves as "swimmers' shampoo"—most of them also contain sulfates. Instead, remove chlorine by cleansing hair immediately after swimming with a sulfate-free cleanser or conditioner. Massage it in and rinse. Then apply another layer of conditioner, combing it through the hair with your fingers. You can either leave it all in if you are sitting by the pool or on the beach, or rinse just some of it out by cupping your hands together under the running water and tossing it over the head. (Those with very fine curls should rinse it completely to avoid weighing the hair down.)

• If you're unable to rinse your child's hair immediately after swimming, put conditioner in a spray bottle and bring it to the pool or beach to spritz in your child's hair each time he gets out of the water. That is better than letting the pool or salt water sit in the hair for a few hours before you can co-wash.

FINDING THE KINDEST CURLY STYLIST

One of the biggest complaints I hear from curlies around the world is "I can't find a stylist to cut my curls or child's curls properly." And if you or your child have had a devastating curly haircut in your past, you both are probably afraid to sit in just any stylist's chair. But that doesn't surprise me. When it comes to curls, beauty school curricula are outdated and vastly unsustainable. However, because there are more naturally curly-haired people in the world than people with naturally straight hair, I believe that cosmetology schools must begin to focus on curls, their organic nature, and their

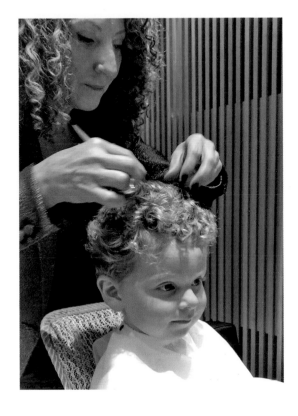

interaction with atmospheric conditions, so hairstylists can learn to cut and care for them accordingly. Until that happens, here are some things to consider before you let anyone approach your child's hair (or your own) with a pair of scissors.

The surest way to find someone who cuts curly hair correctly is to see a haircutter's work. So when you spot someone with curly hair that looks wonderful, ask her where she gets it cut. (Don't hesitate because you think it's intrusive; most people will be flattered.) Social media is another place where hairstylists showcase their craft. Otherwise, keep asking around until you find someone whose curls you relate to. Next, email or call the salon and ask the following questions:

- Is the stylist versed in cutting curly hair?

- Has he or she taken curl classes to advance his or her understanding of curls?

- Has the stylist heard of the CG Method?

- Does the stylist have naturally curly hair? Does he or she wear it curly? If so, that's a good sign; if he or she blow-dries it straight, use your curl instincts and discretion to decide if this person is right for you and your child.

- Will the stylist see your child for a free consultation? That shouldn't be a deal breaker, but it's worth asking. Some places may charge for this service.

- Does the salon offer the option of drying the hair under hooded helmet dryers and with diffusers rather than with blow-dryers and brushes? If not, insist that you want to keep your child's hair curly and just leave with it wet.

- Does the stylist cut curly hair while it's dry? If the answer is no, is he or she willing to be open to this approach? If you get another no, hang up the phone and find a stylist who *does* cut hair dry. This is a must for curly, coily, kinky hair.

- What products does the salon use? If they contain sulfates and silicone, bring your favorite conditioner with you and politely say that you prefer it. Most stylists won't object, especially if your child's hair is in good condition. If the stylist hesitates, tell them your product is doctor recommended. Remember it's *your* child's hair and you are its guardian for a short time.

- Ask how their approach to curly hair is different from their approach to straight hair. If they say they "thin out" or "de-bulk" curly hair, beware. You need gravity and the weight of the original curl formation to give hair its definition.

- Ask if they use a razor to cut hair. Some stylists use them to cut curls, but they aren't as sharp as scissors, so they can create badly torn and frayed ends.

Curly Kid Inspiration

Emma McCoy

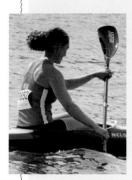

How could I make both my hair care and my sports life (as an elite-level kayaker training for the 2024 Olympics) uncomplicated? I've always wanted my hair to be unapologetically me—bouncy, sassy, sporty, and curly. I agonized over it before walking out the door, and it was never right. At practice, I didn't give it a second thought; I'd just pull it back in a ponytail and keep going. But after practice, my roots would be stretched flat and my curls would be limp, which would only fuel the cycle of frustration and indifference.

I hated my hair in athletic pictures. This was especially true when I was racing in Poland in September 2018 at an international regatta, where there were cameras everywhere. Sprint kayaking at that level means there are 1,001 other things to think of, so I just pulled my hair back in the morning. But when I saw the pictures that were taken, there wasn't a single one I liked. Although I don't think about my hair while exercising, I'm much more confident when my hair looks like me.

Matching my hairstyle to my lifestyle isn't easy, but the CG Method streamlines the process. And that included Lorraine. I went to her for a cut. I didn't know what I wanted. I simply told her to do what she thought best. I sat in shock as she cut off way more hair than I was prepared to lose. The courage it takes me to be successful in kayaking was the same courage it took me to sit in the chair and trust Lorraine. Everyone needs to take a leap of faith; you'll at least learn something and be further along than you were before.

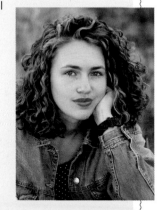

Now it doesn't matter if I'm at school or practice; my hair always looks like me and I'm ready for everything.

• Let's assume you got all the right answers and have made an appointment. But if, when you arrive, your child is told to change and get her hair shampooed, a "bad hair" alert bell should go off. Instead, the stylist should sit you and your child down, examine her hair, touch it, talk with you about it, and then ask what you envision having done—all before picking up the scissors. The stylist should know to pull a typical curl down to its farthest point to see how tight the curl is. If your child's curls vary in tightness, show her which ones have a smaller spring factor. This is important so that she doesn't cut too much. Finally, explain that you'd rather leave the hair a bit too long than too short. Ideally, after cutting the hair dry, the stylist should wet your child's hair and let it dry to see if any remaining hairs need to be trimmed.

TOP SALON CRIMES COMMITTED AGAINST CURLY GIRLS AND GUYS

SLICING, CARVING, THINNING OUT, RAZORING, OR DE-BULKING. Since curly hair has a low molecular weight, razoring and thinning out curls deform the actual curl structure and make the ends look torn, frizzy, and weak. This changes the curls' intrinsic shape as they grow out. Curls rely on a sharp scissor and a clean cut so the haircut lasts longer and the ends look healthy.

TEXTURIZING makes no sense for curls, which are *all* texture and nothing *but* texture! All this does is distort the most natural formation of your child's unique curl shape.

TWISTING requires a lot of work—and, once again, disturbs and distorts your child's curls. Sure, it's gentler than using a curling iron, but it also interferes with the hair's natural state of grace. Some twisting techniques may look lovely on children, but they can take hours to do.

CUTTING YOUR CURLY KID'S HAIR

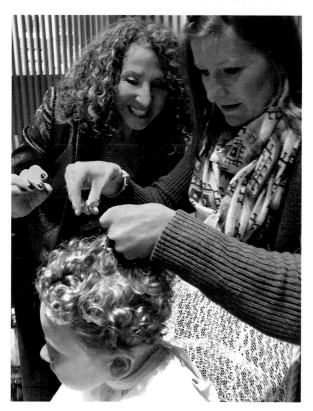

Cutting a very young child's hair is tricky if you're not a trained hairdresser. It can also be tricky for those who *are* trained, because the scissors are very sharp on a moving target, especially toddlers! However, throughout the years many moms and dads with curly kids have asked me to teach them self-*mane'tainance*, and I understand why. After all, bad haircuts are probably the most traumatic memories in a curly girl's or boy's hair history, my own included. When it comes to cutting curly hair, I always say, "It's not what you take off; it's what you leave on." Depending on your spring factor, if you cut an inch off curly hair, it can look like you cut off three or four inches. By now you know that curly hair fibers can fray easily, and as a result, they not only need to be delicately cared for, but also cut with caution. That said, if you stay within these suggestions and logical curl guidelines, you'll be fine!

The most important thing I want to teach you is how to trim, or do what I like to call "oxygenize," your child's precious locks. You can do this if your child needs just a trim, between regular haircuts, to save time and money. To oxygenize

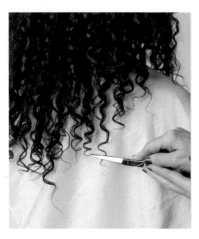

means to refresh and aerate. It also means that you're cutting off the least amount of hair. When the hair is cut, it automatically opens up to the environment. It allows each hair strand to breathe in more oxygen and moisture, and it really makes a difference. I think of it like trimming plants or grass in the garden. The forces applied that make continuous healthy growth possible are cutting, watering, and fertilizing, which is the equivalent of conditioning.

I am not talking about cutting off big chunks of hair or totally reshaping it. That's a job for a trusted stylist. I'm talking about a fraction of an inch, half a C curl or at most a full C curl. It will make a big difference when you remove frayed, spidery knots that feel like sugar granules right at the very ends of the hair. With a pair of sharp, professional hair scissors, a small snip can go a long way for curly hair.

THE OXY-TRIM

Think of a beautiful bonsai tree. Your eyes naturally gravitate toward the end of each stem or branch, and you want to cut off any part that looks gnarly and dried-out. By clearing and pruning the plant or tree in this manner, you're helping it take in oxygen and water the moment it is cut and exposed to the atmosphere. As a result, it immediately looks healthy and is ready for new growth. If you apply this thinking to the ends of your hair or your child's hair, you will be amazed at what a difference a little oxy-trim can and will do—especially if your idea is to grow the hair.

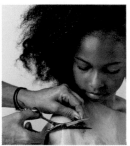

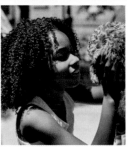

Curly Kid Inspiration

Denise McCoy

My hair was full, thick, and wavy until I hit puberty. My mom did a great job caring for it. I didn't have my curls yet, so she brushed it and I could wear pigtails, ribbons, ponytails, and barrettes. It was wonderful. But when I was eleven years old my mom died. My hair became curly when I hit puberty and no one knew what to do with it. From then on, my hair felt like something I always had to tame, manage, cajole, and "deal with." I tried everything from horse shampoos to mousse to hard, crunchy gels, but nothing really helped.

Then one day, my cousin called to tell me about a coworker's hair transformation. She and her coworkers used to talk about this gal's unruly curly hair, until one Monday when she came in with a mass of glorious curls! My cousin immediately asked her what she had done and passed on what she learned about the CG Method to me. Of course, I dove in headfirst to learn all I could. I also found Lorraine and went to see her. That was about fifteen years ago, and my curls have never been the same! Finally, I learned to love, care for, nourish, and feed them. Now, all these years later, my curls are my shining glory.

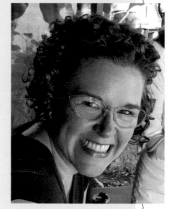

When my daughter, Emma, hit middle school and puberty took over full force, her curls starting coming in. She wasn't very interested in styling her hair, and I didn't push it. I just kept reiterating the importance of good care. She's seventeen years old now and about to embark on her own life journey apart from me. Each day she grows more confident in her curls and how to care for them, what they need, and how to get them to do what she wants. She's proud of her hair and loves it when people ask her about her curls.

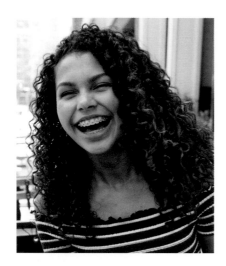

Before doing anything, it's important to buy a pair of high-quality scissors made specifically for hair. These usually cost upward of $100 at a beauty supply store. (If you have a trusted stylist, you can ask her what type of scissors she uses.) They are pricey, but remember, your child's hair is priceless and worth the investment. Please refrain from using scissors made for fabric or paper. The blunt shears won't give hair a clean, sharp cut. In fact, these and other inferior scissors can actually fray the ends, because they tend to be duller than professional hairdressing scissors. The wrong pair will make a gnawing, clinking sound and will often require you to cut the hair a couple of times to get through it. In contrast, a high-quality pair

THE CASE AGAINST EXTENSIONS

Extensions are pieces of extra hair—either real hair or synthetic fibers—that are sewn onto your existing hair. Not only is this process pricey and time-consuming, but it's also not good for the hair and scalp. Some people incorrectly believe that extensions are "protective hairstyling," but that is a myth. The weight of the extensions tugging on your real hair can cause hair thinning, hair loss, and a receding hairline. This creates a vicious cycle where you continue to get extensions to cover up thinning natural hair, which continues to get even thinner—a cycle you don't want to start in childhood, or ever. To make matters worse, many people treat the extensions the same as they treat real hair—with sulfate-filled shampoos and heat styling. Yes, heat styling! Also, extensions can fall out at the most inopportune times. It's just not fun when someone has to say, "Excuse me, miss. You dropped your hair," and trust me, I have observed this many, many times!

Advice from a Stylist

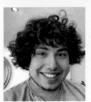

Fabian Bine, owner of Curl Love in Hampshire, United Kingdom

For as long as I can remember, I had my hair cut short because it was easier for my parents to manage. As a teenager, I decided to grow my hair long. I was told countless times, "You look like a mop." One time, a teacher said, "Cut your hair. It looks ridiculous. You're a boy." I was speechless.

Growing up, I was told that people of Asian heritage could not have curly hair. I didn't even know that my own mother was a curly girl in denial when I was growing up. (She is now openly curly.)

Around the age of fourteen, I had an "aha" moment with a friend who told me about wavy and curly hair and said that mine might actually be curly instead of the messy frizz it appeared to be. That night, I scoured the internet and discovered "scrunching." I used a floor fan heater as a makeshift diffuser with no products, and afterward my hair fell into ringlets. I pestered my parents to get me a silicone-free conditioner because I had also stumbled upon the CG Method online. Soon my hair quickly settled into the curl it is today. I am now at a stage where I don't worry about what my hair decides to do. I am happy to follow its lead. A little frizz is a good thing. After all, they say the taller the hair, the closer you are to heaven.

I went into my current salon mad about curls, always encouraging my clients to wear their hair curly. Many people traveled great distances to see someone who knew what they were doing with curly hair. My boss eventually took a class in curly hair too. I am very lucky to have been working in such a supportive environment.

Curly Kid Inspiration

AJ Grovert

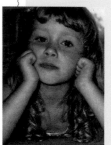

I've always had curls that I saw as beautiful, but the adult women around me struggled with them while I was growing up. After my parents divorced, when I was eleven, I lived with my curly-haired dad. In my early teens, he remarried. My stepmother has straight hair and thought I should have the same. She was always trying to make me and my hair into something we weren't. At their wedding, I wore my hair in a tight ballerina bun, because I knew she wouldn't accept my natural texture in wedding photos. She constantly wanted to blow-dry and straighten my hair, and I let her just to keep the peace. She would try to style my hair the same way she did hers, but while hers would lie flat, I turned into a frizz ball. I got married when I was thirty-one, and the day of my wedding, after I'd had my hair styled naturally, my stepmother asked me if I had a hairbrush. "Not for years," I answered.

My mom, who loves my natural texture now, didn't understand that a curly daughter might have hair needs that were different from the ones she had. Embracing my hair as an adult is like a homecoming. People like my stepmother will always think natural curls look messy. But I've really grown to love my curls, and I'm proud to have inherited them from my dad. He's an example in a lot of things, and this is no exception.

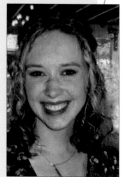

of scissors will seem to silently melt through the hair, cutting it with precision and accuracy. Scissors also come in right-handed and left-handed styles, so make sure to buy the correct one for you and ensure that they are comfortable to hold. Don't use them for anything other than hair, and store them safely between trims. (They're very sharp, so don't leave them around for children to find.) A high-quality pair will last a lifetime and will stay sharp, since, unlike salon scissors, which are used on hundreds of heads per month, they're being used only on your hair and/or your child's. You also don't want to use a pair of thinning shears or a razor, because these will fray and split the ends of the hair.

When it comes to cutting curly hair, I always say, "It's not what you take off; it's what you leave on."

Never cut your child's hair while you're in the dark, in a moving vehicle, or drinking (unfortunately, this happens!). Also make sure you have plenty of time; when you're rushed, you're more likely to make mistakes. And be careful. High-quality hairdressing shears are very sharp, so it's easy to snip your fingers along with your child's hair. Another important note: Don't pull the curls taut when you cut them, because curls are longer when you pull them, so you risk snipping off too much hair. For looser curls, you can see exactly where they lie and what you're going to cut off. You still have to hold them firmly to get a clean line, but do so gently without over-pulling. One exception is fractal curls in their resting state. These can appear to be as short as your child's chin at rest, but way past her shoulders when pulled straight. However, if you cut a fractal curl in its natural resting position, you risk taking off too much. You have to pull it down to its farthest point to just make a teeny, tiny snip at the end.

First, carefully examine your child's natural hair wave or curly terrain. See how it falls around the face and in the back of the head. Ask yourself these questions:

• Are the curls/waves weighed down?

• Is the crown flat?

• Do you see varying curl types or similar textures?

• Are the curls on the bottom very tightly coiled or are they loose?

• Are the curls at the temples tighter or much looser?

• Do the bangs or fringe have tighter or looser curls?

TRIMMING THE ENDS

• Lightly spritz the hair with distilled water, lavender water, or Co-Wash in a Bottle (see the recipe on page 170).

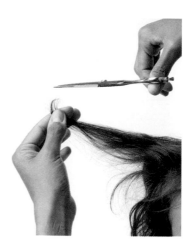

• Open up the curls by placing your splayed hands at the roots and gently shuffling them. This allows the curls to separate and settle into their natural positions. After doing this, you might want to have your child look up to the ceiling and gently shake her head back and forth.

• If the hair is shoulder length or longer, have your child stand up while cutting so you can see how the hair falls naturally. When your child is sitting down, her hair may appear longer than it really is, or she may sit unevenly.

• Look carefully at the overall hair and then the ends, and decide where and how much you plan to trim.

• With your thumb and index and middle finger, take your first "curl unit" and hold it so that the bottoms of your fingers hit where you plan to trim the hair.

• Make sure you're holding the scissors comfortably. From a very young age, we know how to pick up a pair of scissors and use them for cutting paper. Simply pick them up like that.

• Continue to do the same on each curl unit in the hair on that side of your child's head, trimming off equal amounts of hair on each one. Avoid combing or running your fingers through the hair, because this will disrupt and distort the curls' intrinsic shape.

- Next, trim the hair on the other side of the head in the same manner.

- Place your splayed hands on your child's scalp and gently shuffle the hair at the roots. Then look at how each curl falls.

- When you trim your child's bangs or fringe, observe how and where the hair falls, and while it's in its natural position, snip the hair to the desired length.

- Note any stray hairs or uneven, looser locks, and give those a snip the same way. If you are nervous about taking off too much, wait until after you co-wash the hair. If any curl is left behind, it usually shows itself after it has been cleansed, combed through with conditioner, and the hair has dried.

With time, experience, seeing how your child's hair dries after cleansing, and observing it in motion, you will start to have a natural curl instinct. You might even become a curl-cutting expert.

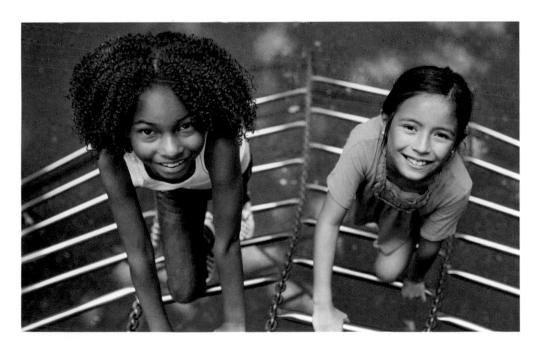

ALL HAIL THE PONYTAIL!

Ponytails are the easiest and most versatile of hairstyles. They keep hair off the face and lift it off the neck, are cool in hot weather, and elegant when styled well. They can also express playfulness or seriousness.

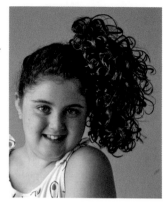

As I've said earlier, but will repeat here because it's so important, ponytails should never be super tight. Ponytails where the hair is pulled back really tautly are not only uncomfortable and can lead to headaches, but they also can actually cause the hair to break off. In severe cases, like when tight ponytails are done frequently, the hairs don't grow back and cause the hairline to recede. Choose soft, fabric-covered ponytail holders, not ones with metal on them as these can saw the hair and cause breakage and damage. And never, ever use an actual rubber band. These can really rip, tear, and damage hair. Decorative ponytail holders are fun, but just make sure there isn't a place for the hair to get tangled.

If you want to spritz the hair before gathering it into a ponytail, Co-Wash in a Bottle is perfect for this. (See the recipe on page 170.) It's also great for spritzing on the finished ponytail to scrunch it into shape. Low ponytails are great for helmets, and a little Co-Wash in a Bottle is useful to help curls bounce back into shape when the helmet comes off.

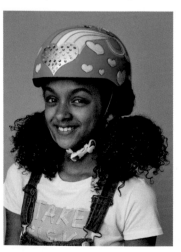

Top ponytails can be embellished with a headband or scarf and are also a great style when your child is wearing a visor. If the hair is long, make a loose bun by pulling the hair only partway through the second time you loop the ponytail holder around it. You can also wrap a section of hair around the ponytail holder to conceal it and give a more natural look. Top ponytails are fun too and are ideal for keeping hair healthy and tangle-free while sleeping.

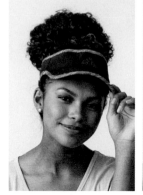
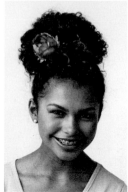

SIMPLE BOX BRAIDS

Simple box braids look great, keep hair off the face, and can stay in for up to a week, so they save time on daily cleansing and styling. Just make sure not to pull braids too tightly as this can damage the hair and over time can cause the hair to break off at the scalp, creating a receding hair line. Wendy Pimentel, a curly hair expert and hairstylist, demonstrates braids on her son Kamerin on pages 150–151. "I like braiding my son's hair for easy maintenance when it comes to morning routines and school," she says. "As a working mom, every minute counts in the morning, and braids keep his hair neat and knot-free."

• Cleanse or co-wash and detangle hair according to the CG Method.

• After detangling, you can leave in a slight residue of the conditioner according to the curl type you're dealing with.

• If you are using a styling agent, make sure it's 100 percent alcohol- and silicone-free. Apply the product to the hair right before starting the braid. I advise using as little as possible. Wearing braids is a great opportunity to detox the hair from too much product. Also the hair will dry faster.

• Use a tail comb to part the hair into rows according to the look you are trying to achieve. You can do rows of hair from front to back or side to side. Try to make your rows evenly spaced and not so tight that the scalp looks pinched or overexposed.

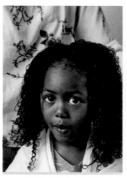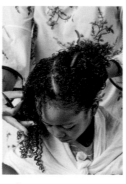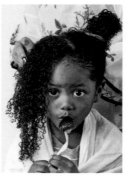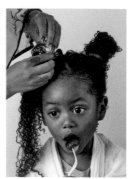

- Use small gummy hair elastics, sometimes called snag-free elastics. They are small, thin, flat rings that lay flat against your hair and hold small amounts of hair securely. They often come in different hair colors or are clear, to disappear into the braid. Twirl the gummy elastic around the very end of the braid to secure it.

- If the hair starts to become dry or tangled as you braid, use a little of the Co-Wash in a Bottle (see page 170) to keep the hair soft and manageable.

- Divide the first row into subsections. Take one subsection and divide it into three sections. Hold two sections with one hand and the third section with the other hand.

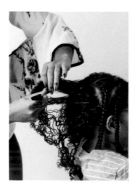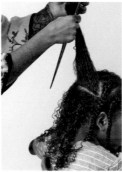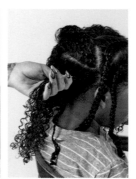

- Take the section of hair on the far right and cross it over the middle section and the move the middle section to the right, creating a braid.

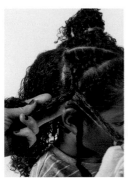 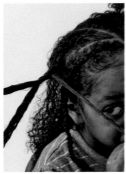 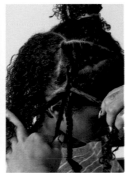

- Cross the section on the left over the middle, and move the middle section to the left. Repeat until you have braided the entire section.

- Repeat on each separate section that you are braiding.

- Twirl the ponytail holder around the braid.

These braids can stay in for a week. For sleeping, wrapping them with a silk scarf keeps them in place and looking their best.

SIMPLE, ROMANTIC TIE-BACK

This is great for longer hair.

- Lift your child's hair up and take two sections of hair, one from each side, close to the nape of the neck.

- Bring both pieces of hair out to the side and then behind the head.

- Tie the two pieces together as in the first step of tying shoelaces. Pull them gently to secure.

- For a simple look, secure the hair with bobby pins that are the same color as your child's hair.

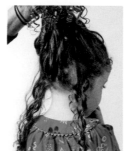
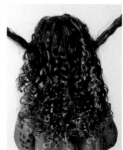
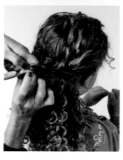
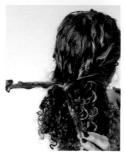

- To add a little more personality or for special occasions, add a decorative barrette or bobby pin.

- If needed, spritz the hair with Co-Wash in a Bottle (see page 170 for the recipe) or just water and scrunch to maintain the curls' shape.

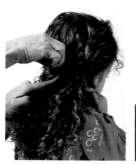
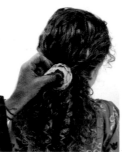
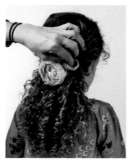
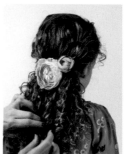

ELEGANT EVERYDAY PULL BACK

- Gather hair in the back of the head. Leave out a section on the front right side of the head.

- Gently put the hair in the back into a ponytail and secure it with a hair tie.

- Take a small section of the hair you left out and twist it up and back toward the ponytail. Secure it with a bobby pin near the ponytail.

- Continue doing this until you've twisted back the entire section of hair that you left out.

- Leave a small curl in front if desired.

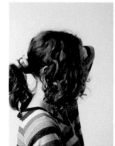
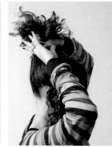
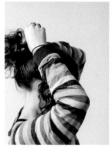
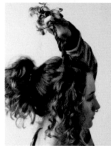

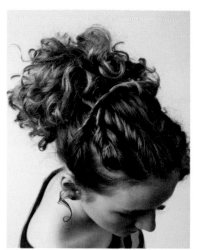
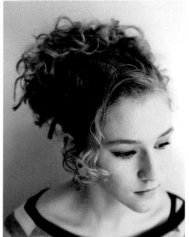

CASCADING PONYTAIL

- With the hair down, take the top section of hair into your hand.

- Secure the hair with a fabric ponytail holder.

- You can leave the hair down in back or pull it back and secure it with one ponytail holder or two.

- If you want to wear this hairstyle with a visor, put on the visor first and pull all the hair through. Proceed to tie the hair.

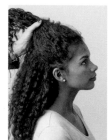
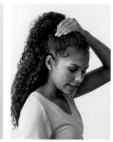
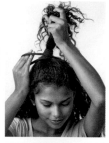
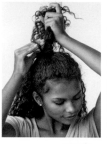
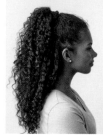
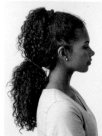
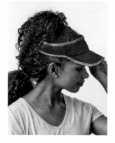
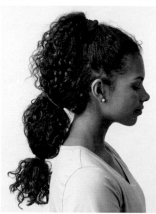

SPORTY TIE-BACK

- Gather the hair at the back of the head while leaving out a small section on one side of the front of the head.

- Secure the hair in a ponytail holder.

- Take the section of hair that you've left out and twist it.

- Bring the twisted section out to the side.

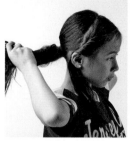 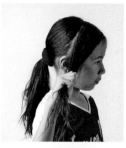 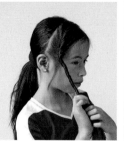 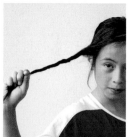

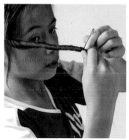 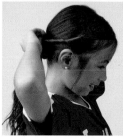 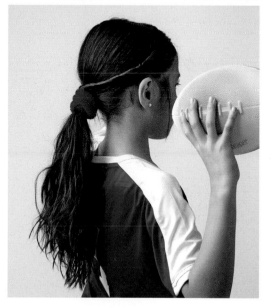

- Place a bobby pin at the end of the twist.

- Secure the twist with the bobby pin near the back of the ponytail.

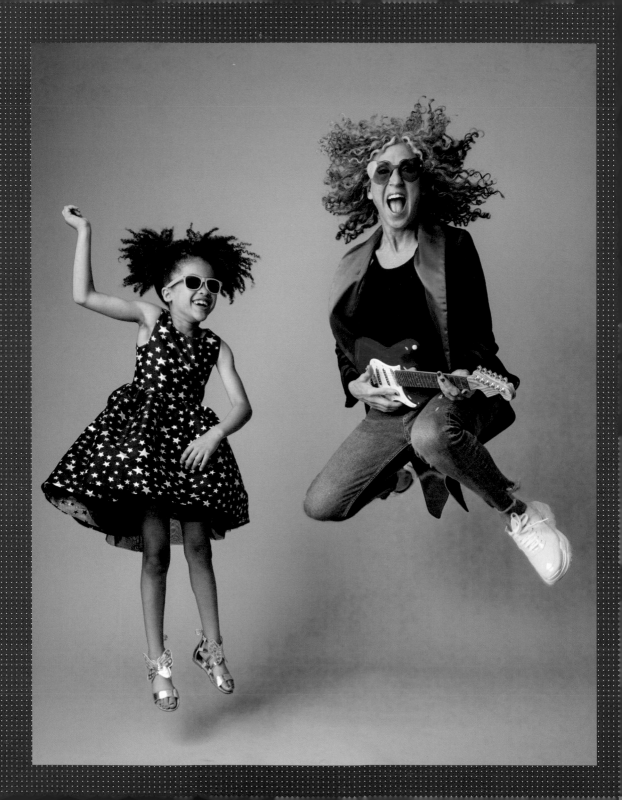

Six

All-Natural Homemade Recipes & Remedies

Curls don't need to be anything other than themselves, and neither do you.

'I've always loved making my own hair and skin potions from natural ingredients. Your skin is your largest organ—and that includes your scalp! Whatever you put on your skin is absorbed into your body, so make sure you know what you are consuming! Following are some natural, simple, fun, and inexpensive do-it-yourself recipes that all ages can benefit from. And they'll leave your hair looking and smelling lovely.

Mist in You
Lavender All-Purpose Herbal Cleanser

Lavender has many well-known therapeutic qualities—its scent alone is soothing. It calms the nervous system and can help relax even the jumpiest of kids. I have a pot of this mist steeping on my stove at all times, and my very active four-year-old grandson loves to open the lid and breathe it in. He calls it lavender juice! It also acts as a natural disinfectant. In French, *laver* means "to clean or to wash." It can be used in spray form to refresh, cleanse, and deodorize the hair and scalp.

INGREDIENTS

1 large, lidded stainless steel pot—ideally one used only for this purpose.

½ gallon (8 cups) water

5 to 10 drops of the purest form of lavender essential oil you can find. True essential oils evaporate in your hands after you rub them in and leave behind a refreshingly pleasant scent with no oily residue.

3 empty spray bottles (available at most drugstores or health food stores)

1. Fill the pot with the water.

2. Cover and bring to a rolling boil for at least 10 minutes to get rid of impurities. (Check occasionally to make sure too much water isn't evaporating.)

SPRAY IT WITH LOVE

Lavender spray makes a wonderful gift for friends, whether they have curly hair or not. Once you get hooked on the spray, you'll find lots of other uses for it. Some of my clients have told me they took it to the delivery room when their children were born and instructed their husbands to spray it on them during labor for a calming effect. You can also use it as a room, closet, or car deodorizer. It eliminates unwanted odors and is much healthier than aerosol sprays, filled with numerous toxic chemicals that we—and especially our young ones—do not need to be breathing. You can also spray it on bed linens to help you drift off to sleep or on clothes in the dryer. Another use is for refreshing your hair, face, and clothes after you've been cooking. A 3-ounce travel size is a must for your carry-on when you travel by air so you can spritz it while on the plane.

3. Remove the pot from the heat and immediately add the lavender oil. Stir, and replace the lid so the lavender infuses the water. Let sit for at least 3 hours, the longer the better.

4. Fill the spray bottles with the cleanser. Store at room temperature or in the refrigerator.

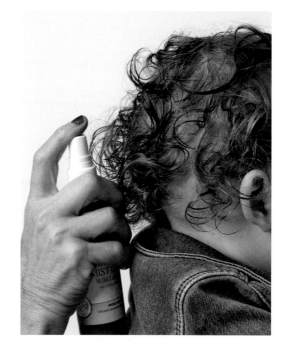

Wipe Right
Cleansing Wipes for Scalp, Hair, Face, Hands, and Body

The chemicals in many traditional baby wipes are far from natural. Your skin does not need that type of chemical stripping, whether or not you are a baby. What irritates me (pun intended) is that big brands are still not telling us the whole truth about what's in their products. A common ingredient is bronopol, a preservative also known as 2-Bromo-2-nitro-1, 3-propanediol. It releases formaldehyde as it breaks down, is a known irritant, and really shouldn't be used in baby products or human products—period. Another dangerous ingredient that wipes may contain is phthalates, which have been linked to everything from asthma to infertility. Say no to that stuff!

INGREDIENTS

25 bamboo cloths cut into wipe-size squares (If you want to use biodegradable baby wipes, simply rinse them in hot water to rinse away the scent and chemicals, then squeeze them out to dry.)

2 cups plain boiled water or 2 cups boiled water with 3 to 4 drops of apple cider vinegar or 2 cups lavender-infused water from the Mist in You recipe (see page 158)

A bowl large enough to hold the wipes and water

1 large plastic ziplock bag

1. Place the cloths or wipes in the bowl and soak in one of the following:

- fragrance-free boiled water

- apple cider vinegar water

- lavender-infused water from the Mist in You recipe

- water with a different essence that your child likes, such as rosemary, light rose, lilac, or clary sage

2. Place wipes into a ziplock bag.

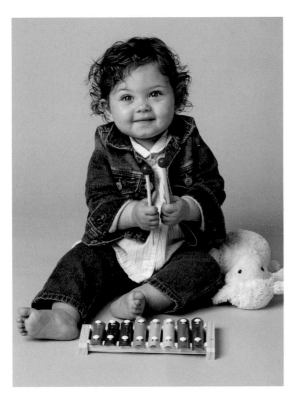

These wipes are a staple in my bag for an array of on-the-go activities. When your child is hot and bothered, gently graze a towelette over their hair or use it to scrunch and refresh their curls. I use the wipes on my scalp after a workout and on my hair after I've been cooking, and I add gel to them to help tame a halo of frizz.

What Knots?

A Daily Co-Wash Detangling Spritz

This is great for everyday use on knots or matted hair, or to spot cleanse and refresh on days you don't co-wash.

INGREDIENTS

2 cups boiled water or 2 cups water infused with 5 drops of lavender, rose, rosemary, or clary sage essential oil

½ cup silicone-free, water-soluble conditioner

1 quart-size jar with a tight-fitting lid

2 small or 1 large spray bottle, depending on your preference. You will have about 9 ounces of product.

1. Combine all the ingredients in the jar.

2. Shake the mixture vigorously until it looks milky. If the solution separates, the conditioner may have silicone, oils, or butters in it. That isn't ideal, but if you shake it well before each spritz, it'll be okay.

3. Pour the solution into the spray bottles. Store in the refrigerator or at room temperature.

TO DETANGLE

• Isolate the knot and spritz the What Knots? spray into it.

• As the knot absorbs the milky conditioner, gently begin to pry open and separate the hair strands, releasing the knots.

• You may need to spritz several times to soften the strands before finger-combing the knot out. Once the knot is detangled, scrunch up the hair, then repeat on remaining knots.

Ginger Ninja Rinse

Ginger has a long history of medicinal use in China, where people drink ginger tea for colds, the flu, and other ailments. It acts as an analgesic and antioxidant, it stimulates the immune system, and it can help alleviate nausea. It also can be used for sunburn or as a scalp, hair, and full-body rinse after you've spent time in the sun, salt water, or chlorine. If you'd like enough to use as a body splash, double the recipe.

INGREDIENTS

1 cup water

1 thumb-size portion of frozen ginger root
(2 ginger teabags can be used as an alternative.)

1 fine grater

Silicone-free conditioner

1. Bring the water to a boil. Grate the frozen ginger root with a fine grater. Add it to the pot of boiling water, where it will melt in. If you're using teabags, add to the water and let steep for at least 10 minutes.

2. Allow the mixture to cool before pouring it over the hair and massaging for 2 to 5 minutes.

3. Rinse the hair and follow with a silicone-free conditioning co-wash. Allow the conditioner to be absorbed, detangle the hair with your fingers, and then rinse.

Sugar Babes

This recipe is great for cradle cap; a dry, scaly scalp; or dandruff. It works for all ages!

INGREDIENTS

½ cup fine brown sugar

1 cup silicone-free conditioner

1 12-to-16-ounce sterilized glass jar or clean, recycled jam jar with lid

1 plastic cup, scoop ladle, or watering can

1. Combine the ingredients in the jar. Mix well for about 3 minutes. Before giving your baby a bath, apply Sugar Babes to the scaly or dry area and gently massage it in using a circular motion with one or two fingers.

2. Tilt your baby's head up and thoroughly rinse with warm water using a plastic cup, scoop ladle, or watering can.

3. For thick or long hair, follow with a little more silicone-free conditioner and comb it through with your fingers. Rinse out all the conditioner or leave some in for more curl definition.

Teens and adults suffering from mild eczema or really dry skin on the scalp, body, elbows, and feet can benefit from this recipe too. Simply apply Sugar Babes to the dry area, massage in for a few minutes, and rinse it off using a circular motion. Do not follow with soap as it will further dry out those areas. Store any leftovers in a sterilized glass jar or a recycled jam jar with a lid.

Rocka'bye Cradle Cap

Green gram, also known as Moong Dal, is a small green bean grown in India. When ground up, it is a wonderful natural treatment to help heal cradle cap. It can be found in Indian food stores, health food markets, and online.

INGREDIENTS

3 tablespoons green gram flour

1 to 2 tablespoons spring water or distilled water

1 small sterilized mixing cup or bowl

Diluted silicone-free conditioner

1. Combine all the ingredients in a mixing cup until they become a paste.

2. Apply the paste to your baby's scalp 10 minutes before bath time, rubbing it gently into the scaly areas only.

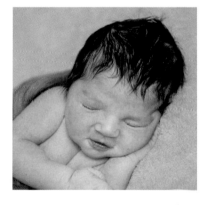

3. Wait 10 minutes, then gently rinse. If your baby has a lot of hair, follow with a diluted silicone-free conditioner and then rinse again.

Soothing Sage, Lavender, and Nettle Tincture

This tincture is great for itchy scalps and as a hair deodorizer for after cooking or just as a freshener. It's also great for eczema, dry patches, or dandruff and as a follow-up and/or preventive lice treatment.

INGREDIENTS

¼ cup dry nettle leaves

¼ cup dry sage leaves

1 12-to-18-ounce canning jar

1½ cups witch hazel

2 to 5 drops of lavender or rosemary essential oil (or the oil of your choice)

1 coffee filter

1 12-ounce dark glass bottle with dropper, available at most drug, craft, and health food stores

1. Place the dry nettle and sage leaves in the canning jar and add the witch hazel and essential oil.

2. Let it steep for 1 to 4 weeks. The longer the better, as steeping will extract the components from the herbs.

3. Strain the mixture through a coffee filter and squeeze out all the goodness. Dispose of the leaves.

4. Transfer the mixture to a glass bottle with a dropper.

5. Refrigerate, as coolness adds to the soothing effect.

6. Before bed or on a non–co-wash day, apply 1 to 3 full droppers to the scalp. Massage in for a couple of minutes and blot excess with a paper towel. Do not rinse, brush, or comb the hair; instead, allow it to air-dry. Avoid getting the tincture into the eyes. If you do, rinse the eyes with cool water.

OTHER USES:

• Apply to blemishes or oily T-zones.

• Add a few drops of sweet almond oil to use as a face cleanser. Apply it to the skin and wipe it off with a cotton ball and splash rinse.

• Apply it to dry patches on the elbows or knees.

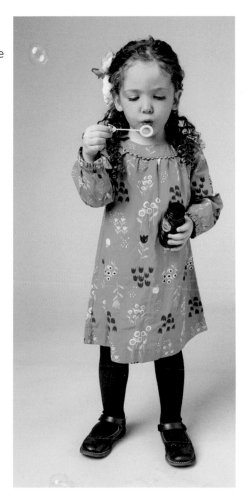

Halo Goodbye Hair Gel

This easy-to-make product is great for all curl types and hair with a high frizz factor.

INGREDIENTS

¼ teaspoon clear unflavored gelatin or pectin

½ cup hot water

¼ cup aloe vera pulp or pure aloe juice

2 tablespoons coconut water
(more for stronger hold)

1–3 drops lavender essential oil

A few small, sterilized jars for storage, or one large enough to hold a bit more than a cup of product

1. Pour the gelatin or pectin into a bowl and add the hot water, aloe vera juice, coconut water, and essential oil. Whisk slowly to combine the ingredients.

2. Let the mixture cool. Once cool, it should have the consistency of hair gel. Transfer to a jar or other container. Keep refrigerated and use within a year.

TO USE: After cleansing, scoop about a tablespoon of the Halo Goodbye Hair Gel into the palms of your hands, rub your hands together lightly, then evenly distribute over the hair canopy. Either scrunch upward to capture curl forms or glide fingers downward to elongate curls. Use more if necessary. Shake curls into their natural positions. If you choose, clip or pin hair at the roots for extra height and do not disturb until dry.

Silicone Valley

This is a fresh and gentle way to remove silicone buildup from your hair. Apple cider vinegar on its own is very acidic, so in order to use it on your hair and scalp, neutralize its pH with conditioner.

INGREDIENTS

1–2 tablespoons apple cider vinegar

¼ cup silicone- and sulfate-free cleanser or conditioner

1. Add the apple cider vinegar to the cleanser or conditioner. How much you use depends on the length and thickness of your hair.

2. Apply the mixture to wet hair, making sure no curl is left behind, and let it sit for 10 to 20 minutes.

3. Rinse your hair thoroughly.

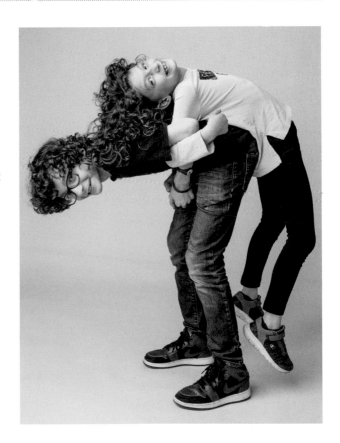

Co-Wash in a Bottle

Throughout the book, I've mentioned this Co-Wash in a Bottle and its many uses. It can be used as a leave-in styling product if your or your child's hair doesn't feel hydrated enough after co-washing. It can also help tame frizz or refresh hair on days when you're not co-washing. Just spray it in and scrunch.

INGREDIENTS

¼ cup silicone- and sulfate-free conditioner

¾ cup distilled water, spring water, or water that's been boiled and cooled

8-to-12-ounce spray bottle

Combine conditioner and water in a spray bottle. Shake well before each use. You can also use the Mist in You water in place of the distilled water for a scented variety.

Scrunch-ees

You can make your own curl-loving hair bands, which are not only fun and original but also help prevent frizz and breakage. All you need are stockings or tights—opaque ones, sheer ones, or fishnets (which are great because the hair can breathe).

• Cut a leg off the hose and then cut it into horizontal strips, making them as wide or as narrow as you want.

• Cut off the elastic waistband, which can be used as a headband on dry hair anytime or, when hair is wet, to keep it off your or your child's face. Use the same way you would use any elastic headband.

Curly Kid Inspiration

Kirsty Allford

As a child, I was desperate for curls. I couldn't do anything with my thin, poker-straight hair. Even a ponytail wasn't an option, because elastic bands would just slide out. To make matters worse, my cousin had the most beautiful curls, and I was jealous both of her hair and of all the attention she got for it. Now, my five-year-old daughter, Bae, has stunning ringlets. For as long as she can remember, her hair is what people comment on as soon as they meet her, so from a young age, she's been very aware that it's different. Most of the time she's really proud of her curls, but if they don't fall how she hoped they would (and let's face it, curls have a mind of their own!), she throws some pretty hefty tantrums.

Bae is too young to understand hair straightening, but she sometimes wishes her hair wasn't as curly. She doesn't see many people with curls in real life, so I feel fortunate for social media. I show her pictures from Instagram accounts like Lorraine's, among others. For Bae, seeing so many strong, positive female role models exuding self-confidence and proudly showing off their hair in its wild, natural state has stopped her from feeling self-conscious and really helped her to see just how special her "crazy, beautiful hair" (as she calls it) really is.

This influence is remarkable: Bae started kindergarten recently, and each child had to introduce themselves and say their favorite thing about themselves. Bae's reply? Her hair, of course!

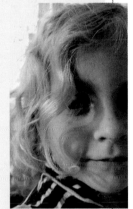

Kirsty's daughter Bae

Curly Kid Inspiration

Shillo Beaton

My mum blows out her straight(ish) hair, so she never understood curly hair. Growing up, I longed to have her brush my hair and experience the intimacy I saw between other mothers and daughters; instead, my hair was a battle between us. I spent my childhood with her wetting it and scraping it back into bunches every morning. If I cried—and we all know the pain of having your ears and eyebrows brushed—she said, "If you cannot handle it long, you can have it short." I spent my childhood with my hair going from short to midway down my back and then short again.

At school I always had a fear of the lice nit nurse. When she came, she took out my hair bands and as she examined every part of my scalp, my hair grew and grew. Afterward, I'd try to wrestle my wild hair back into a ponytail or some sort of bun. On those days, my classmates called me names like "Brillo pad" and "pube head." When I got to high school, I soaked my hair every morning and added handfuls of gel. I clipped the front bit back and left the rest down. I pretty much kept that style until recently.

My hair was one of the "imperfections" I hated about myself—the kind you hold deep and don't speak about often but that weighs heavy on your soul each day. Other curlies would share a sympathetic look with me at times, knowing the pain. Straight-haired people would comment on how lovely my curls were, yet I could never accept it.

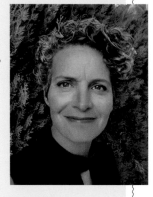

My relationship with my hair changed when it turned gray. I liked it and felt that I should let it bloom! That led me to the CG Method, then to *Silver Hair: A Handbook*, and the icing on the cake was the best-ever curl-by-curl cut last year. My advice to my younger self and any kids who dislike their curly hair today is to learn the CG Method and whisper to yourself that curly hair is the best hair. If you follow the method, you'll know it's true.

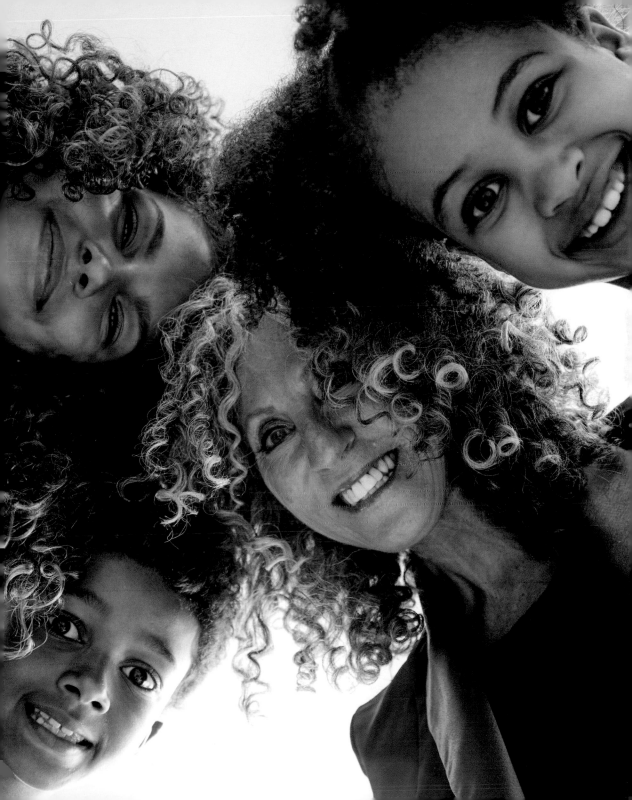

Curly Girl Method Terms and Conditions

THE CG METHOD™: "Curly Girl/Guy Method," a term that's used globally in the curly community. This simple and logical approach to curly hair care replaces poor habits like shampooing with sulfate-filled products and using heat-styling tools with healthier, more sustainable daily hair-care habits, such as cleansing and conditioning with 100 percent sulfate- and silicone-free products.

CG APPROVED, CURLY GIRL/GUY APPROVED: Products that are approved to be used with the CG Method. For example, CG Approved cleansers don't contain sulfates and approved conditioners are free of silicones, heavy oils and butters, parabens, and fragrances.

CLEANSING: The term used in the CG Method instead of "shampoo" or "wash." It's the use of a sulfate- and silicone-free cleanser or conditioner combined with gently massaging the scalp with your fingertips to stimulate the scalp and remove any dirt, oil, or product residue. This method of cleansing the hair avoids harsh detergents that dry out the hair.

CO-WASH: The CG Method term for "conditioning wash," or using a 100 percent sulfate- and silicone-free conditioner to cleanse, hydrate, detangle, and organize curls.

CURL BY CURL™ CUTTING: The method of cutting hair that focuses on cutting curls dry and in their natural state, addressing each curl individually.

DRY CUTTING: The method of cutting hair dry.

OXYGENATING/DUSTING THE ENDS: To trim the very end of each hair strand to allow it to "breathe in" oxygen and receive maximum moisture from conditioning. A sure sign the hair is ready for a trim is when it begins to knot at the dry ends more than usual.

GEL CAST OR PRODUCT CAST: The result of a gel or styling application that has fully dried and casted the curls into their natural form, leaving the curls frizz-free and crystallized.

PINEAPPLE: A simple high ponytail at the top of the head, where the gathered strands are pulled through a hair tie and the rest is splayed out naturally. This can help preserve curls while sleeping or exercising.

SPLASH, BAPTISM, OR TRICKLE RINSE: A gentle splash of water from cupped hands after cleansing or co-washing to retain some conditioner that is beneficial to dryer hair types; this method also preserves more fragile wave and curl formations that strong water streams can disturb.

SPOT CLEANSING: Isolating and cleansing just an area of the hair that has become frizzy, disbursed, or knotty. This targets just the curls that need help, letting the rest of the hair remain undisturbed. For children's hair, spot cleansing stops one tangle from growing into more.

SPRING-BY-SPRING™ FACTOR: To measure the distance between the length of a curl when it falls naturally in its dry state and the length when the curl is fully extended and stretched to its furthest point. This shows why cutting curls dry is so important to the CG Method—it determines how much or how little to cut off.

Acknowledgments

Thank you to all the wonderful curly kids, big and small, and the amazing parents, guardians, and the passionate curl stylists who shaped, scrunched, and curled this beautiful book. You shared your natural hair stories with sweet and open spirits. We owe many thank-yous to Julio Sandino, Veronica Tapia, Edward Joseph, Rosie de Silva, Vitoria Wense, Shey Aponte, Kazem Naderi, Aaron Anthon, Saulo Galtri, Kristy Wilson, and Viki Mackinder. To Carolan Workman, Susan Bolotin, Anne Kerman, and Becky Terhune at Workman, thank you for helping us create our vision to connect to the curls we are born with. This book is about unlearning, educating, being uncomfortable, and inspiring our curly kids, their parents, and guardians to stand in their naturalness. We appreciate our PR team Rebecca Carlisle, Lathea Mondesir, and Cindy Lee. A special thanks to Mary Ellen O'Neill, our curly compass who once again navigated and guided us through the bends, swerves, and u-turns to create *Curly Kids*, a book we are proud to share with the ever-expanding, hypo-galactic curly world. Thank you for being such a great midwife, pushing us in all ways to do better, with hardly any labor pains. Many thanks to Lucy Schaeffer for the fabulous photos.

LORRAINE'S ACKNOWLEDGMENTS

It has been a privilege to work alongside Michele Bender again. You truly complete me in this realm, and I am looking forward to *Curly Girl*, the sequel.

Kaih, Shey, Dylan, Veronica, Silas, and Venaih, you are the loves of my life. I thank you for your unwavering support.

To all the Curlies I have had the opportunity to meet, listen to, and learn from, it has been incredible to witness all of your curl journeys and transformations, both near and afar and how the grassroots movement of one Curly telling another is the only reason I am here and yes, you all could have written this book! I want to say thank you for also being an inspiration for others by simply being your beautiful, authentic selves and standing your natural ground.

MICHELE'S ACKNOWLEDGMENTS

Lorraine, what I have learned from you over these last ten years about curls, kids, and life is hard to put into words, and I am so grateful for ALL of it. This is our third book together, and I look forward to many more! Lily and Jonathan, thank you for being rays of sunshine in my life and for giving me the best job of all. Thank you to Jon for patiently listening to all things curly and being such an amazing source of love and support. Melissa, Zoe, and Judy, most people are lucky if they have one best friend. I am beyond blessed to have three. To Mom, Mort, Todd, and Vivien, you are the best family anyone could ask for.

About the Authors

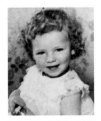

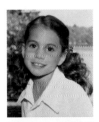

LORRAINE MASSEY, a pioneer in the booming Curly Girl movement, created the CG Method, which has since been adopted by hundreds of stylists worldwide. At the beginning of her career, Lorraine introduced the No(Sham)Poo ideology to the curl world, offering a sulfate-free alternative to shampoo. Today, Lorraine is the sole owner of Spiral (x,y,z), a multidisciplined salon; and founder of CurlyWorld, a line of haircare products. Lorraine spends her days teaching the Curl By Curl method to stylists worldwide. *Curly Kids* is her third book, following bestsellers *Curly Girl: The Handbook* and *Silver Hair: The Handbook.*

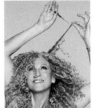

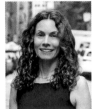

MICHELE BENDER is an award-winning freelance book and magazine writer. She coauthors and ghostwrites books with high-profile experts and celebrities as well as proposals. Some of these bestsellers include *Believe Me* by Yolanda Hadid, deemed one of the "100 Best Memoir Books of All Time" by BookAuthority, and *The Immune System Recovery Plan* by Susan Blum, MD, a leader in functional medicine. Michele and Lorraine also worked together on *Curly Girl: The Handbook* and *Silver Hair: The Handbook.*

Give Your Hair the Love It Deserves
with Lorraine Massey

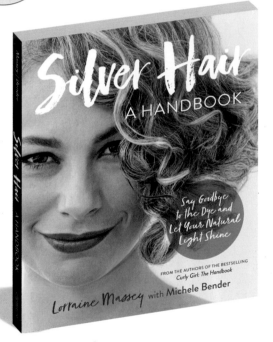

OVER 500,000 COPIES IN PRINT!

EXPANDED SECOND EDITION

curly girl
THE HANDBOOK

A CELEBRATION OF CURLS

- Daily Routines for Different Curl Types
- Lorraine's "No More Shampoo!" Epiphany
- Trimming Your Own Hair
- Plus Q's & A's

by Lorraine Massey with Michele Bender

Silver Hair
A HANDBOOK

Say Goodbye to the Dye and Let Your Natural Light Shine

FROM THE AUTHORS OF THE BESTSELLING Curly Girl: The Handbook

Lorraine Massey with Michele Bender

Celebrate the beauty of curls in this buoyant how-to manifesto and curly girl support group in one.

Learn how to grow out your color and love your gorgeous, naturally silver hair.

Available wherever books are sold, or visit workman.com.

workman